Imaging of Foreign Bodies

Antonio Pinto · Luigia Romano
Editors

Imaging of Foreign Bodies

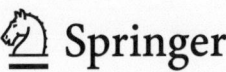

Editors
Antonio Pinto
Luigia Romano
Department of Diagnostic Radiological Imaging
Cardarelli Hospital
Naples
Italy

ISBN 978-88-470-5859-0   ISBN 978-88-470-5406-6 (eBook)
DOI 10.1007/978-88-470-5406-6
Springer Milan Heidelberg New York Dordrecht London

© Springer-Verlag Italia 2014
Softcover reprint of the hardcover 1st edition 2014
This work is subject to copyright. All rights are reserved by the Publisher, whether the whole or part of the material is concerned, specifically the rights of translation, reprinting, reuse of illustrations, recitation, broadcasting, reproduction on microfilms or in any other physical way, and transmission or information storage and retrieval, electronic adaptation, computer software, or by similar or dissimilar methodology now known or hereafter developed. Exempted from this legal reservation are brief excerpts in connection with reviews or scholarly analysis or material supplied specifically for the purpose of being entered and executed on a computer system, for exclusive use by the purchaser of the work. Duplication of this publication or parts thereof is permitted only under the provisions of the Copyright Law of the Publisher's location, in its current version, and permission for use must always be obtained from Springer. Permissions for use may be obtained through RightsLink at the Copyright Clearance Center. Violations are liable to prosecution under the respective Copyright Law.
The use of general descriptive names, registered names, trademarks, service marks, etc. in this publication does not imply, even in the absence of a specific statement, that such names are exempt from the relevant protective laws and regulations and therefore free for general use.
While the advice and information in this book are believed to be true and accurate at the date of publication, neither the authors nor the editors nor the publisher can accept any legal responsibility for any errors or omissions that may be made. The publisher makes no warranty, express or implied, with respect to the material contained herein.

Printed on acid-free paper

Springer is part of Springer Science+Business Media (www.springer.com)

Preface

Foreign bodies are a frequent and serious problem in emergency departments: ingested foreign objects may occur accidentally or deliberately. Most ingested foreign bodies pass through the gastrointestinal tract without a problem. However, ingested or inserted foreign bodies may cause bowel obstruction or perforation or may lead to severe hemorrhage, abscess formation, or septicemia. Foreign body aspiration is common in children, especially those under three years of age. Chest radiography and CT are the main imaging modalities for the evaluation of these patients. On plain radiographs, metallic objects, except aluminum, are opaque, and most animal bones and all glass foreign bodies are opaque. Most plastic, wooden foreign bodies and most fish bones are not opaque on radiographs; CT is very helpful in these cases.

Key factors influencing patient management include the type of object, its physical characteristics, the location of the object, the time elapsed since its ingestion, aspiration or insertion, associated medical conditions, the presence or absence of symptoms, and evidence of complications.

This textbook will provide an overview related to the critical role of diagnostic imaging in the assessment of patients with suspected foreign body ingestion, aspiration, or insertion.

The 12 chapters present a wide series of cases related to ingested, aspirated, or inserted foreign bodies. In addition, intra-abdominal foreign bodies, intravascular foreign bodies and foreign bodies from penetrating wounds are presented.

We hope that this textbook will provide informations of benefit to Residents in Radiology, Radiologists and Physicians daily involved in the Emergency Department in the management of patients with suspected foreign body ingested, aspirated, or inserted.

October 2013

Antonio Pinto
Luigia Romano

Contents

1. **Plain Film and MDCT Assessment of Neck Foreign Bodies** 1
   Antonio Pinto, Raffaella Capasso and Luigia Romano

2. **Tracheobronchial Foreign Bodies** 9
   Maria Giuseppina Scuderi, Domenico Aronne, Raffaela Giacobbe,
   Paola Martucci, Luciano Biagio Montella, Bruno Del Prato
   and Stefania Daniele

3. **Foreign Bodies of the Gastrointestinal Tract** 25
   Antonio Pinto, Silvana Nicotra and Vincenzo Di Mauro

4. **Intra-Abdominal Foreign Bodies: Gossypiboma and Abdominal Wall Meshes** 37
   Nicola Gagliardi, Nicoletta Pignatelli Di Spinazzola,
   Vincenzo Di Mauro, Giuseppe Ruggiero and Carlo Muzj

5. **Abdominal Compartment Syndrome Due to Hepatic Packing** 47
   Ciro Acampora, Ciro Stavolo and Maria Paola Belfiore

6. **Foreign Bodies as Complications of Biliary Stents and Gastrointestinal Stents** 55
   Antonio Pinto, Daniela Vecchione and Luigia Romano

7. **Intravascular Foreign Bodies** 67
   Raffaella Niola, Sergio Capece, Mario Fusari and Franco Maglione

8. **Foreign Bodies As Complications of Endovascular Devices** 81
   Antonio Pinto, Stefania Daniele and Luigia Romano

9. **Retained Intracranial and Intraspinal Foreign Bodies** 89
   Gianluigi Guarnieri, Luigi Genovese and Mario Muto

| 10 | **Role of Magnetic Resonance Imaging in Diagnosing Foreign Bodies**... | 101 |

Rosaria De Ritis, Francesco Di Pietto and Carlo Cavaliere

| 11 | **Soft Tissue Foreign Bodies**............................. | 105 |

Antonio Pinto, Amelia Sparano and Mario Tecame

| 12 | **Foreign Bodies and Penetrating Injuries**.................... | 115 |

Giorgio Bocchini, Giacomo Sica, Franco Guida, Luigi Palumbo, Sujit Vaida and Mariano Scaglione

Index 127

Plain Film and MDCT Assessment of Neck Foreign Bodies

Antonio Pinto, Raffaella Capasso and Luigia Romano

1.1 Introduction

Foreign body (FB) aspiration and ingestion represent the main source of foreign bodies located in the neck. In children, the aspiration of foreign bodies most often occurs between the ages of 1 and 3 years, and the aspirated object is most commonly found at the level of the right main stem bronchus [1]. Less often, foreign bodies become lodged in the upper airway (most commonly the vallecula, epiglottis, vocal folds, and subglottis) [1]. Peanuts, seeds, and beans represent the foreign bodies most commonly aspirated [1].

In adults, patient groups at risk of FB ingestion include those intoxicated, those undergoing dental surgery, the visually impaired, and those with bulimia nervosa who accidentally swallow an object that is used to induce vomiting. Of the FBs brought to the attention of physicians, 80–90 % will pass through the gastrointestinal tract spontaneously; however, 10–20 % will require endoscopic removal and about 1 % will require surgery [2, 3]. Moreover, FBs that are large, long, sharp, or irregularly shaped tend to cause complications.

A. Pinto (✉) · L. Romano
Department of Diagnostic Radiological Imaging, Cardarelli Hospital,
Via A. Cardarelli 9, 80131, Naples, Italy
e-mail: antopin1968@libero.it

L. Romano
e-mail: luigia.romano@fastwebnet.it

R. Capasso
Department "Magrassi-Lanzara", Second University of Naples, Piazza Miraglia 2, 80138, Naples, Italy
e-mail: Raffaella85@libero.it

Perforation of the pharyngeal or esophageal wall represents a possible complication, and migration of the FB in the adjacent tissues can be facilitated by swallowing, coughing, and esophageal peristalsis, as well as by the weakening of the pharyngeal wall due to the local inflammation. FBs in the hypopharynx and esophagus almost always need radiological evaluation to demonstrate the type of the FBs and its location, and the presence of any underlying esophageal conditions [4].

1.2 Pharyngeal Foreign Bodies

Most ingested FBs do not become impacted in the oropharynx. The most common exceptions are fish or chicken bones, although any sharp or irregular object may become impacted [5, 6]. These objects most often lodge in the soft tissue at the base of the tongue, but may also be found in other areas, such as the tonsil or pyriform sinus [5]. Fish bones, particularly, most commonly lodge in the oropharynx, especially the tonsillar fossa and posterior third of the tongue. Localization of bones in these areas is relatively straightforward using pharyngeal mirrors or flexible nasopharyngoscopes. It is when impaction occurs at less common sites, such as at the cricopharyngeus or cervical oesophagus that radiological investigation has a role to play.

Patients usually know exactly when the object became impacted: typically, they present to the emergency department with an FB sensation and odynophagia several hours after ingestion, and they may have attempted one or more home remedies, such as drinking fluid, eating bread, or trying to grasp the object with their own fingers [7]. Hypopharyngeal FBs can be detected with a good physical examination and an indirect laryngoscope examination. However, most of the FBs are located in cervical esophagus, where they cannot be detected, and then the otolaryngologist must search for additional information from radiology or endoscopy [8].

1.3 Upper Esophageal Foreign Bodies

The cervical esophagus is a common site of FB impaction: anatomic features of the esophagus are important to identify because there are areas that are at risk of FB impaction. The first area is located posterior to the cricoid cartilage, at the level of the C6 vertebra, where the esophagus begins with the upper esophageal "sphincter" or cricopharyngeus muscle. The upper esophageal sphincter is the most common site of impaction in pediatric patients. The second is at the level of T4 where the distal aortic arch descends posterior to the midesophagus [9]. Distally, there is also an area of narrowing at the lower esophageal sphincter (LES). Many materials can lodge in the esophagus; they can be classified as food bolus impactions or true FBs. True FBs can be subdivided into blunt objects, sharp objects, and miscellaneous (narcotic packs and disk batteries) [10]. The most commonly encountered upper esophageal FBs include dental work, coins, bones, and fruit pits. Other frequently encountered objects in children include crayons, marbles, small toys, keys, stones, and safety pins. There is also a geographic and cultural influence on the type of FB ingested.

1.4 Role of Imaging in the Detection of Pharyngo-Esophageal Foreign Bodies

The first diagnostic tool for the evaluation of patients with suspected pharyngo-esophageal FBs is radiography. Anteroposterior and lateral neck, anteroposterior and lateral chest, and abdominal radiographs should be obtained. The radiological visualization of a FB depends on its radiopacity [11]. FBs in the esophagus are much more likely to be radiopaque. Coins (Fig. 1.1) are the most commonly impacted object in children. The visibility of a fish bone (Fig. 1.2) depends on the fish species, location, and orientation; however, the majority is not seen on plain films, with much higher success in the hypopharynx than oropharynx [12]. Many objects, such as meat, tiny bones, aluminum, glass, plastic, and wood, may be radiolucent and not visualized on plain radiographs [4].

Multidetector row computed tomography (MDCT) is very useful for the evaluation of patients with suspected pharyngoesophageal FBs (Fig. 1.3) because it offers short examination time and the ability to obtain diagnostically useful coronal and sagittal reconstruction images. MDCT can detect ingested objects such as slightly calcified objects that are missed by conventional radiographs. Moreover, MDCT is also helpful to detect FB complications (Fig. 1.4), such as perforation, fistula, or abscess [9].

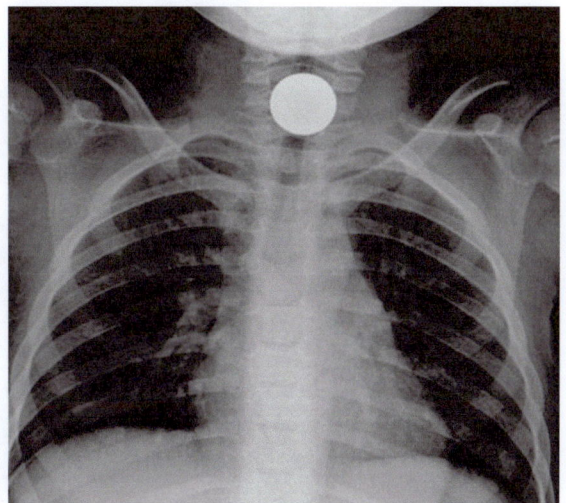

Fig. 1.1 Chest radiograph shows the presence of a radiopaque FB (*coin*) lodged between the hypopharynx and the cervical esophagus

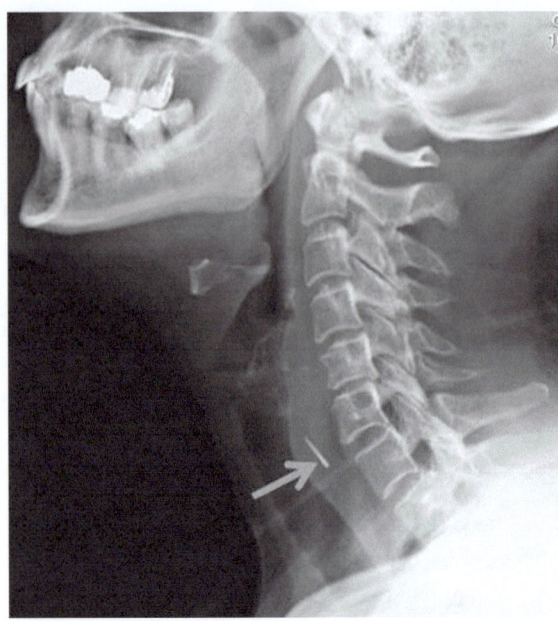

Fig. 1.2 Neck lateral plain film shows the presence of a radiopaque FB (*fish bone*, *arrow*) anterior to the body of C6

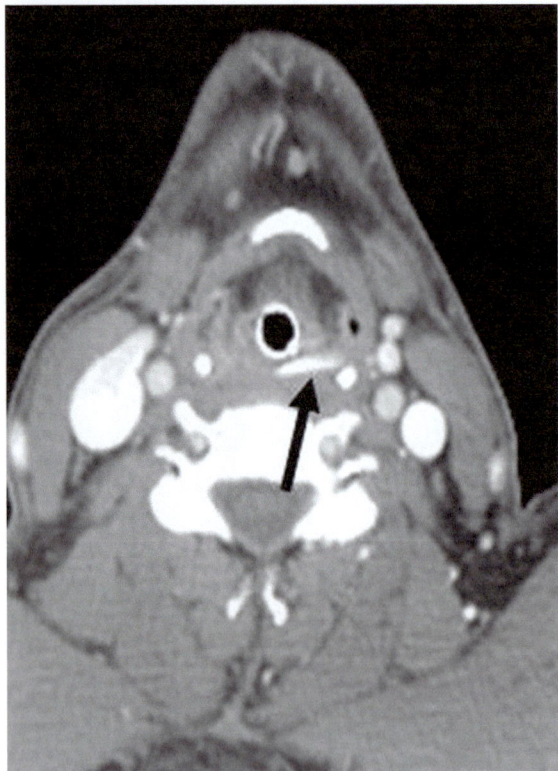

Fig. 1.3 MDCT shows the presence of an impacted hypopharyngeal FB (*fish bone*, *arrow*)

Fig. 1.4 MDCT demonstrates an impacted hyperdense FB (*arrow*) at the level of the hypopharynx with a contiguous abscess

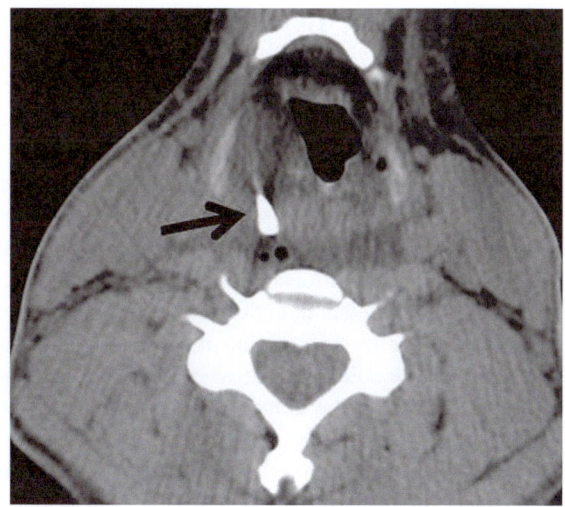

Fig. 1.5 Neck anteroposterior radiograph shows the presence of a linear radio-opaque FB (*needle, arrow*) located in the soft tissues

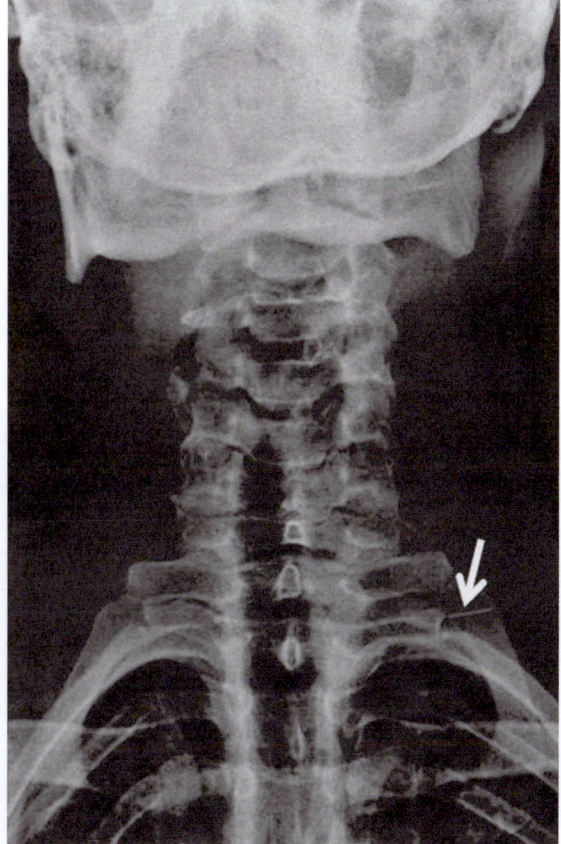

1.5 Neck Soft Tissue Foreign Bodies

A retained FB in the soft tissue of the neck (Fig. 1.5) may determine severe infection or inflammatory reaction: due to this reason, the detection and the removal of the FB is necessary [13].

Bullet injuries can determine the presence of a FB in the soft tissue (Fig. 1.6). Bullets are usually described by their caliber, which is a measurement of their diameter in inches or in millimeters. Although the caliber of a bullet is important, it has only a loose relationship to the weight of the bullet and the size of its charge. These latter parameters help determine the kinetic energy of the bullet, which is an important factor in determining its wounding potential. Bullet injuries are most severe in friable solid organs, where damage may be caused by temporary cavitation remote from the actual bullet track. Dense tissues (e.g., bone) and loose tissues (e.g., subcutaneous fat) are more resistant to bullet injury. Bones modify the behavior of bullets markedly, altering their course, slowing them down, and increasing their deformity and fragmentation [14].

Imaging techniques are required to identify the FB and establish its exact location prior to surgical removal attempt. Radiographic evaluations are routinely performed in order to confirm the presence of radio-opaque foreign bodies in the soft tissues of the neck such as glass, metal, and stone within the soft tissue [15, 16].

Limitations of radiography include non-visualization of radiolucent foreign bodies, radiation exposure and failure of precise localization during removal.

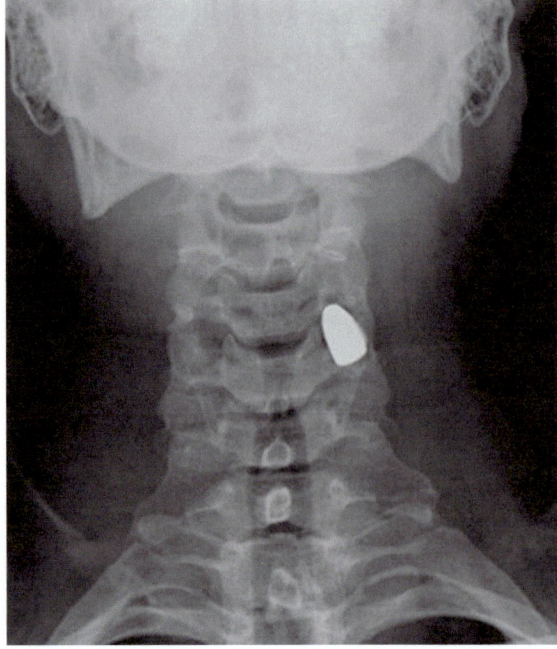

Fig. 1.6 Radiograph of the neck shows the presence of a projectile lodged in the soft tissues

Radioscopy offers a more accurate topographic assessment and allows reference points to be marked on the skin to aid subsequent FB removal. However, radioscopy exposes patient and operator alike to relatively high doses of ionizing radiation.

Ultrasonography is the first choice investigation in the diagnosis of an FB retained in the soft tissues, as it has a sensitivity and specificity of 90 and 96 %, respectively [17, 18]. The limitations of ultrasound are well known: it is an operator-dependent technique and will only display FBs retained in superficial tissues [19].

1.6 Conclusions

FB aspiration and ingestion represents the main source of foreign bodies located in the neck. The diagnosis of unwitnessed FB ingestion can be delayed and complicated, increasing patient morbidity and mortality. The first diagnostic tool for the evaluation of patients with suspected pharyngoesophageal FBs or with suspected neck soft tissue FBs is radiography.

The diagnosis of foreign bodies within the neck, particularly bones can be potentially awkward due to the ossification of the cricoid, thyroid or hyoid cartilages. Lateral neck radiograph may still have a role to play in the investigation of an impacted fish bone in the aero-digestive tract.

MDCT is superior to plain radiographs for the detection of pharyngoesophageal FBs and provides additional crucial information for the management of complicated cases especially related to those which are sharp or pointed.

References

1. Ludwig BJ, Foster BR, Saito N et al (2010) Diagnostic imaging in nontraumatic pediatric head and neck emergencies. Radiographics 30:781–799
2. Binder L, Anderson WA (1984) Pediatric gastrointestinal foreign body ingestions. Ann Emerg Med 13:112–117
3. Velitchkov NG, Grigorov GI, Losanoff JE et al (1996) Ingested foreign bodies of the gastrointestinal tract: retrospective analysis of 542 cases. World J Surg 20:1001–1005
4. Smith MT, Wong RK (2007) Foreign bodies. Gastrointest Endosc Clin N Am 17:361–382
5. Wu IS, Ho TL, Chang CC et al (2008) Value of lateral neck radiography for ingested foreign bodies using the likelihood ratio. J Otolaryngol Head Neck Surg 37:292–296
6. Jones NS, Lannigan FJ, Salama NY (1991) Foreign bodies in the throat: a prospective study of 388 cases. J Laryngol Otol 105:104–108
7. Anderson KL, Dean AJ (2011) Foreign bodies in the gastrointestinal tract and anorectal emergencies. Emerg Med Clin North Am 29:369–400
8. Marco De Lucas E, Sádaba P, Lastra Garcıa-Barón P, et al (2004) Value of helical computed tomography in the management of upper esophageal foreign bodies. Acta Radiol 45:369–374
9. Pinto A, Muzj C, Gagliardi N et al (2012) Role of imaging in the assessment of impacted foreign bodies in the hypopharynx and cervical esophagus. Semin Ultrasound CT MRI 33:463–470

10. Duncan M, Wong RK (2003) Esophageal emergencies: things that will wake you from a sound sleep. Gastroenterol Clin North Am 32:1035–1052
11. Pinto A, Scaglione M, Pinto F et al (2006) Tracheobronchial aspiration of foreign bodies: current indications for emergency plain chest radiography. Radiol Med 111:497–506
12. Lue AJ, Fang WD, Manolidis S (2000) Use of plain radiography and computed tomography to identify fish bone foreign bodies. Otolaryngol Head Neck Surg 123:435–438
13. Mohamadi A, Kodabakhsh M (2010) Wooden foreign body in lung parenchyma, a case report. Turk J Trauma Emerg Surg 16:480–482
14. Pinto A, Brunese L, Scaglione M et al (2009) Gunshot injuries in the neck area: ballistics elements and forensic issues. Semin Ultrasound CT MRI 30:215–220
15. Flom LL, Ellis GL (1992) Radiologic evaluation of foreign bodies. Emerg Med Clin North Am 10:163–176
16. Graham DD Jr (2002) Ultrasound in the emergency department: detection of wooden foreign bodies in the soft tissues. J Emerg Med 22:75–79
17. Jacobson JA, Powel A, Craig JG et al (1998) Wooden foreign bodies in soft tissue: detection at US. Radiology 206:45–48
18. Bray PW, Mahoney JL, Campbell JP (1995) Sensitivity and specificity of ultrasound in the diagnosis of foreign bodies in the hand. J Hand Surg Am 20:661–666
19. Callegari L, Leonardi A, Bini A et al (2009) Ultrasound-guided removal of foreign bodies: personal experience. Eur Radiol 19:1273–1279

Tracheobronchial Foreign Bodies

Maria Giuseppina Scuderi, Domenico Aronne, Raffaela Giacobbe, Paola Martucci, Luciano Biagio Montella, Bruno Del Prato and Stefania Daniele

Any material different from air entering into the tracheobronchial tree, and eventually into the lung, may be considered a foreign body.

We do not consider here the lung injury deriving from inhalation of gas different from air (acute inhalational injury or chronic-inhalational-lung disease) but only injury deriving from solid or fluid materials.

Aspiration occurs when solid or fluid materials, usually from nasal or oral cavity or from oropharynx, pass through the glottis and enter the conducting airways and eventually reach the lung parenchyma. Typically, the Aspiration or Penetration syndrome is characterized from cough, wheezing, dyspnea, and cyanosis. This can be a life-threatening emergency which needs immediate intervention; otherwise it can apparently resolve and go undetected for a long time, also years. The Aspiration syndrome happens more frequently in childhood but it can also be observed in adults. Two peaks of incidence of foreign body aspiration have been observed, the first in the second year of life and the second in the sixth decade of life. [1].

Children in the age range of 1–4 years put everything into their mouth and eventually run with the object in the mouth; in such circumstances sudden sneeze, coughing, laughing, or crying may cause aspiration. Moreover, the lack of molars and premolars determines an "explosive" progression of the alimentary bolus toward the pharynx, favoring inhalation. Vomiting with aspiration of gastric contents frequently occurs in every stage of life. In adult dental procedures,

M. G. Scuderi (✉) · S. Daniele
Department of Diagnostic Radiological Imaging, Cardarelli Hospital,
Via A. Cardarelli, 80131, Naples, Italy
e-mail: margiscuderi@hotmail.com

D. Aronne · R. Giacobbe · P. Martucci · L. B. Montella · B. D. Prato
Department of Bronchial Endoscopy, Cardarelli Hospital, Via A. Cardarelli, 80131, Naples, Italy

situations of impaired consciousness (from drugs, alcohol, anesthesia) and neurological or neuromuscular disease can cause aspiration of foreign bodies [2].

The glottis is the narrowest point of the conducting airways and sometimes larger objects can stop in the larynx and cause strong coughing with spontaneous expectoration or sudden death from asphyxiation.

The position of the body during aspiration can affect the preferential site of localization of the foreign body because the distribution of the material depends mainly on the law of gravity and the anatomical configuration of the airways (Figs. 2.1, 2.2, 2.3, 2.4, 2.5, and 2.6).

When entering in the lower respiratory tract larger and heavier material or fluid should follow the straightest and most gravitary course and should preferentially locate in the right main-stem bronchus or in the right lower bronchus with axis angulated at only 20–30° with respect to the tracheal one compared to 40–60° of the left main stem bronchus' axis.

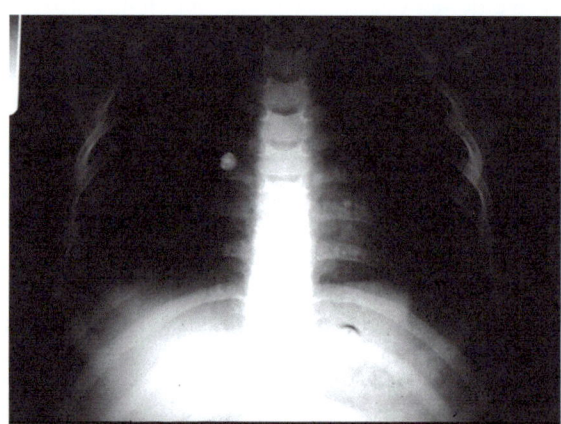

Fig. 2.1 Radiopaque foreign body (stud earring) in right main bronchus

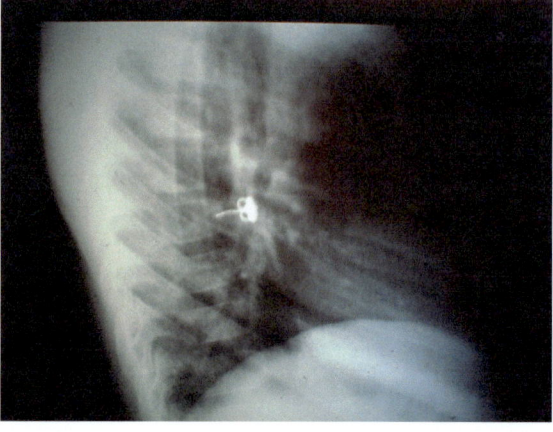

Fig. 2.2 Radiopaque foreign body (stud earring)

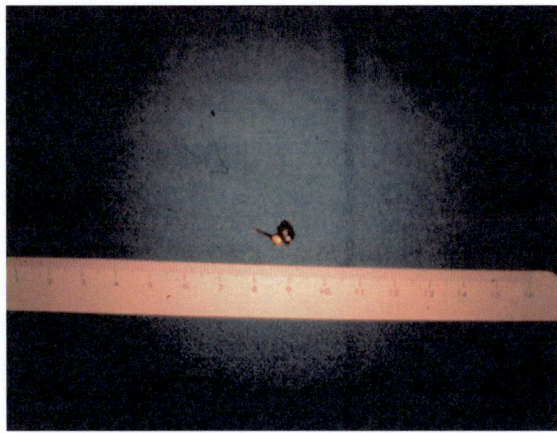

Fig. 2.3 Stud earring bronchoscopically removed

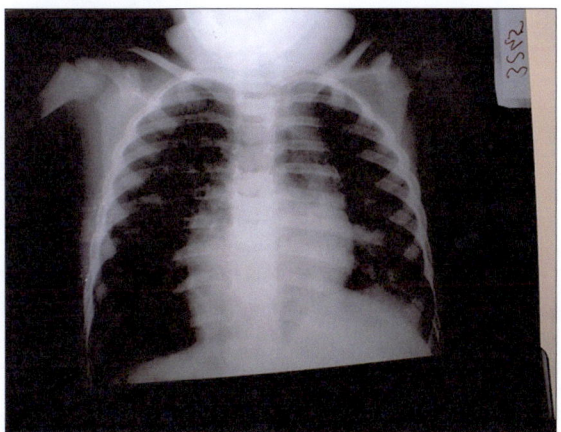

Fig. 2.4 Inspiratory chest radiograph. No evidence of radiopaque foreign body. Hyperinflation of right lung

Indeed, preferential location of tracheobronchial foreign body in the right bronchial tree was demonstrated only for the adult population of a study comparing a child and adult patient population. Moreover, in the child group, foreign bodies were preferentially found in the proximal airways (larynx, trachea, and right and left main bronchi) probably because of their minor caliber [1].

When reaching the lung, finer and more fluid materials preferentially involve, in the supine position, the dependent posterior segments of the upper lobe, and the apical segments of the lower lobe.

In orthostatism, there is the preferential involvement of the basilar segments of the lower lobes and localization is more diffuse as in other areas of the lung (Figs. 2.7, 2.8, 2.9, and 2.10).

In the lateral decubitus, the distribution regards preferentially the apical and posterior upper lobe.

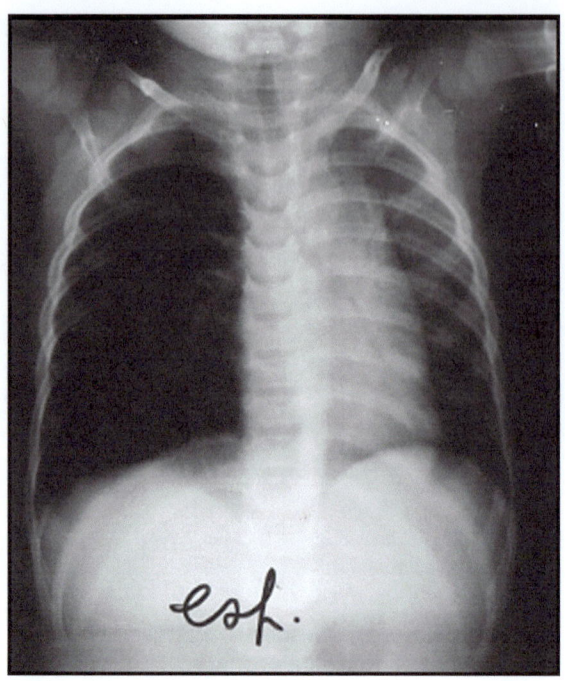

Fig. 2.5 Expiratory chest radiograph: air trapping in the right lung with contralateral mediastinal shift

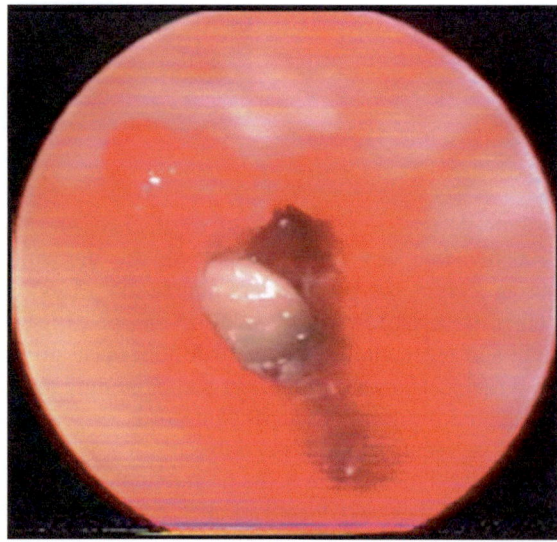

Fig. 2.6 At bronchoscopy food particle obstructing right main bronchus

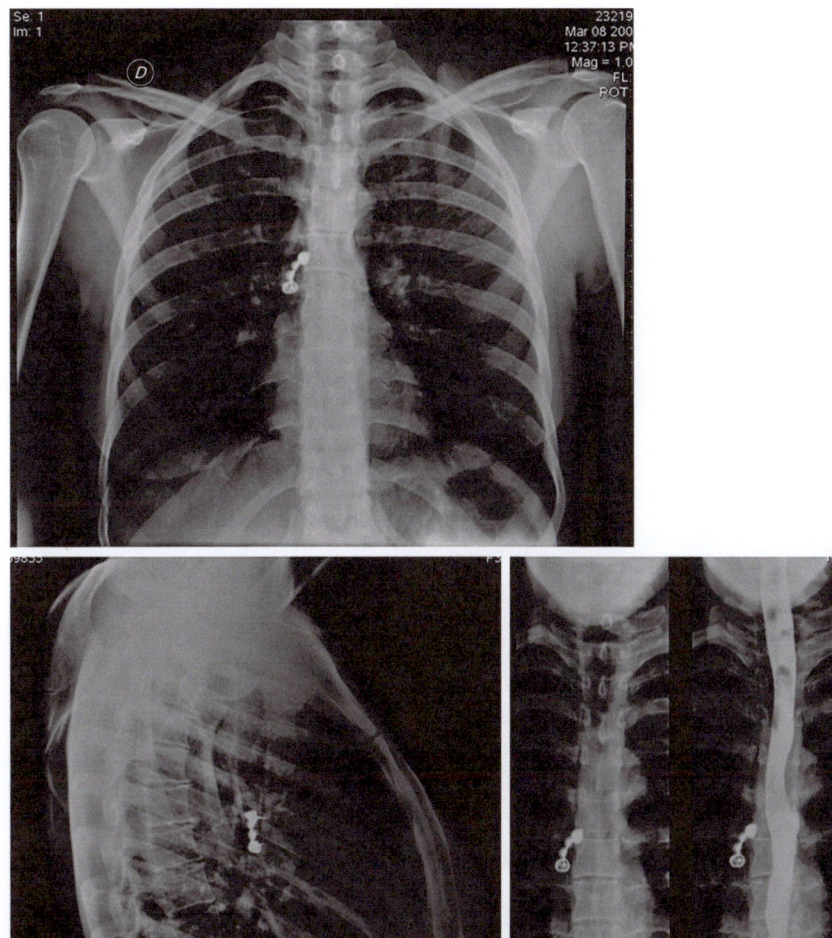

Fig. 2.7 Radiopaque dental bridge (four elements) projecting in the right main bronchus

The anterior portions of the lung are usually involved when aspiration occurs in the prone position, as in near-drowning.

Aspirated material can come not only from external sources but also from inner sources: such as from esophagus or stomach in situations of functional or anatomical defects (tracheobronchial-fistulas). Infective foci of the nasal,

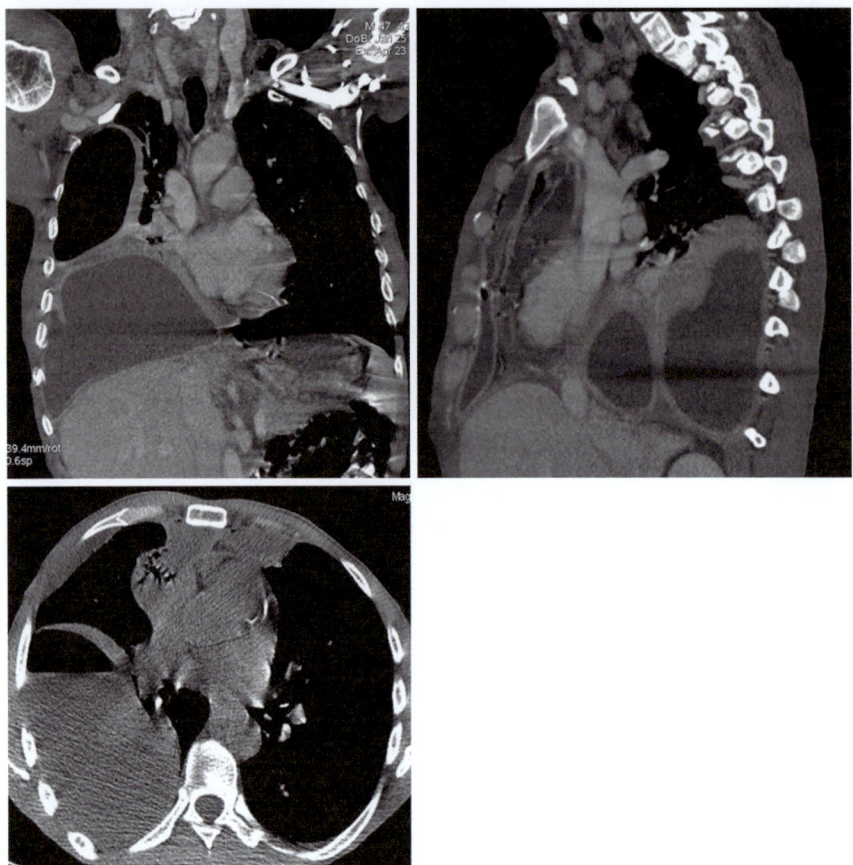

Fig. 2.8 CT performed for mediastinitis in patient with odontogenous abscess. Calcific opacity in the lumen of a segmental bronchi of right lower lobe suspected for foreign body. At bronchoscopy removal of fragment of tooth in B8

oropharyngeal cavity or of the lung itself (cyst or abscess fluid-filled or tubercular cavity) can become another source of aspirate.

A little amount of aspiration of oral or gastric secretions is considered frequent during sleep and anesthesia also in normal adults and is usually not clinically significant.

Nasopharyngeal and oropharyngeal tubes for endoscopy or tracheostomy do not prevent but actually increase the risk of aspiration.

Most frequent aspirated particles are piece of food (nuts, legumens, seeds, fragments of animal bones) and teeth, or little objects or pieces of toys.

The effects of aspiration depend on the amount of aspirated material, the dimensions of the particles, and their chemical nature; they can be acute or chronic.

Fig. 2.9 Wisthler lodging in the left main bronchus (endoscopically removed)

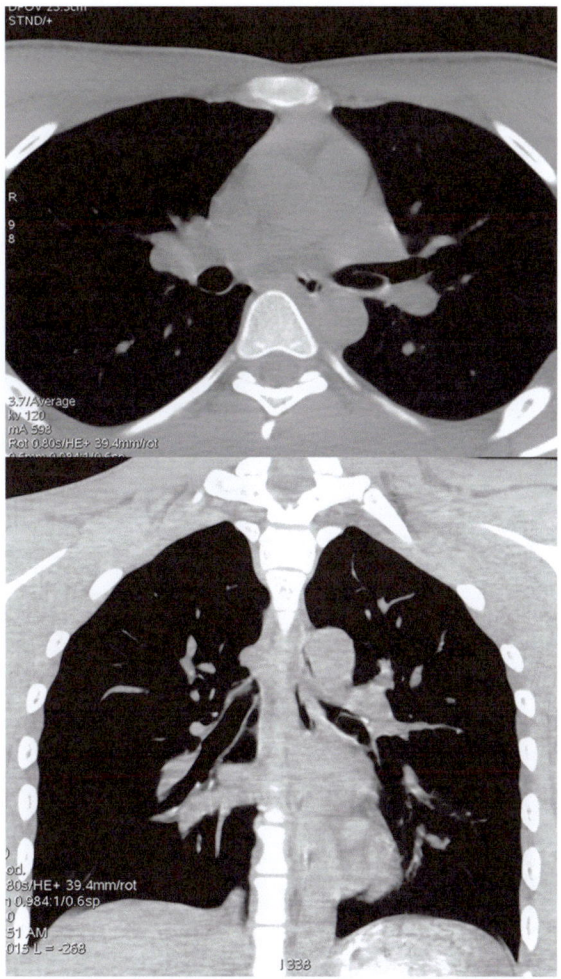

The nature of aspirate can produce different aspiration syndromes:

GASTRIC ACID Acute, massive aspiration of a great amount of gastric acid (pH less than 2.5) is called Mendelson's syndrome and determines in a few minutes an acute chemical lung injury with severe alveolar damage defined as Aspiration Pneumonitis.

Chronic repeated aspiration of small quantities of gastric acid is involved in recurrent pneumonia and chronic fibrosis.

PARTIALLY DIGESTED FOOD and in particular lentils and other leguminous material such as beans and peas can cause a granulomatous pneumonitis called lentil aspiration pneumonia.

Fig. 2.10 Accidental aspiration of gasoline

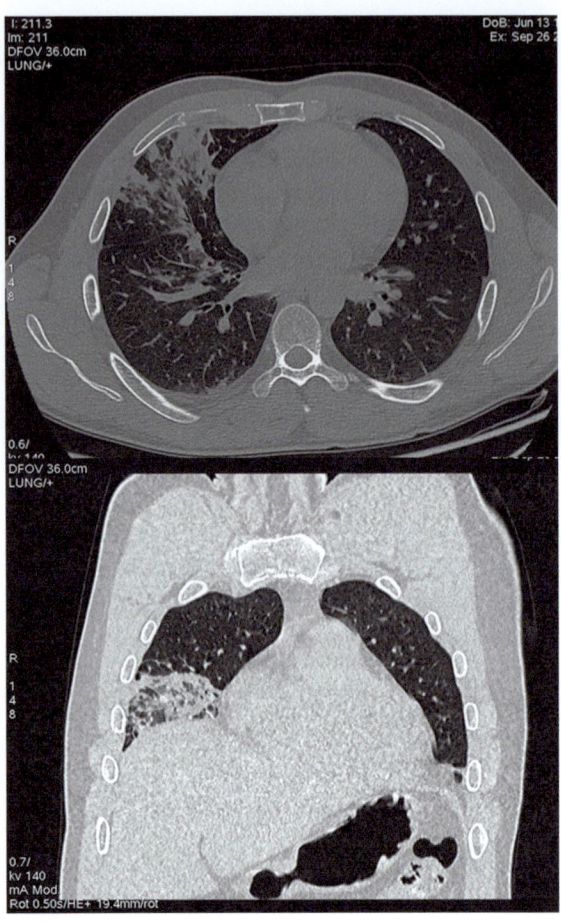

INFECTIOUS MATERIAL from the oropharinx, especially in patients with poor oral hygiene and advanced periodontal disease, can cause an infectious process called Aspiration Pneumonia.

WATER, fresh or salt, when aspirated in great quantity in near-drowning cause pulmonary edema.

SAND or GRAVEL may be aspirated during drownings, surfing accidents, and motor vehicle collisions.

LIGTHER HYDROCARBONS can be aspirated from a person who has siphoned fuel and from fire-eaters.

If aspirated in great quantity they cause a chemical pneumonia called fire-eater pneumonia.

OIL ASPIRATION mineral oil and oily nose drops cause exogenous lipoid pneumonia.

BARIUM ASPIRATION may occur during imaging of the gastrointestinal tract (Fig. 2.11), [3, 4].

Acute complications.

Lodging of aspirated in the trachea causes immediate obstruction of the lumen with penetration syndrome and may require rapid removal by bronchoscopic procedure. Wedging in a main or lobar bronchus may cause total obstruction with atelectasis of the relative parenchyma (lobar or of the entire lung), partial obstruction with hypoventilation (localized wheezing no imaging sign) or, with check valve mechanism, air trapping (also called obstructive emphysema) and eventually pnx and pneumomediastinum.

Wedging in a segmental bronchus in adults less frequently causes complete atelectasis because of the preserved collateral ventilation; in infants atelectasis is more useful because of the absence of the Kohn's pores.

A sharper foreign body (Fig. 2.12) can cause perforation of the bronchial wall and bleeding or can even cause a bronchopleural fistula and pneumothorax.

Foreign body, especially organic or toxic material, acts on the great airways inducing inflammatory effects with edema and acute inflammation, in the parenchyma edema, hemorrhage, pneumonia, and abscess.

Late complications.

Obstruction can later lead to recurrent pneumonia, abscess, and empyema. Prolonged irritation from foreign body with intermittent infections may cause bronchial stricture, localized bronchiectasis, and even hemoptysis (Fig. 2.13).

2.1 Imaging Findings

Imaging findings are not specific and diagnosis is easy only with a known history of episode of aspiration; many cases may initially remain undetected.

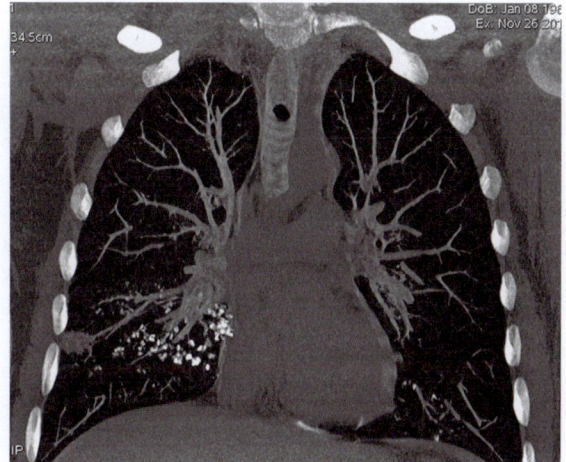

Fig. 2.11 Alveolar hyperdensities from pregressed aspiration of barium

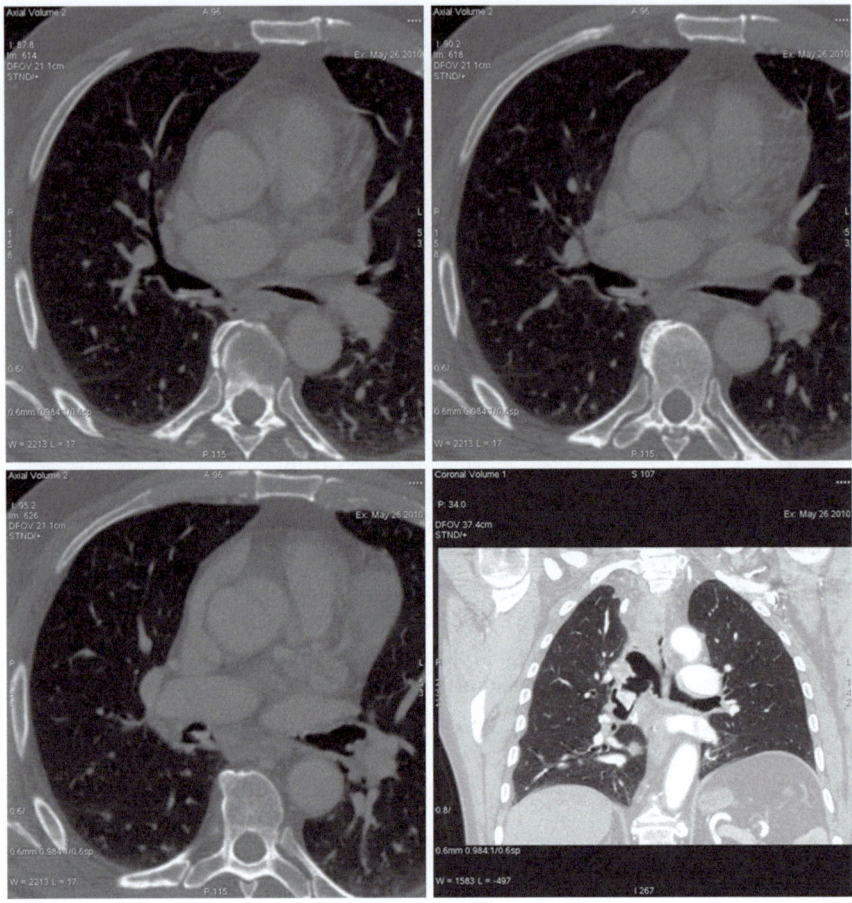

Fig. 2.12 MDCT performed for hemoptysis; foreign body partially obstructing the lumen of right superior lobe and intermediate bronchus in axial plane and in coronal reformatted MIP

Radiographic signs:

Direct visualization of the foreign body; depends on the density of the aspirate and is best for radiopaque material. (Figs. 2.1, 2.2, 2.3, and 2.7).

Chest radiograph may be completely negative especially in case of radiotransparent foreign body (Figs. 2.4, 2.5, and 2.6).

Atelectasis segmental, lobar or of an entire lung (Figs. 2.4 and 2.5).

Obstructive hyperinflation, mediastinal shift (Figs. 2.4 and 2.5).

Air trapping on expiratory chest radiograph or lateral decubitus (Figs. 2.4 and 2.5).

(In infants: in normal conditions dependent lung is less inflated than the contralateral, in case of air trapping dependent lung appears hyperlucent).

Consolidations gravity dependent.

Obstructive pneumonia.

Fig. 2.13 Arterial phase of the previous study; close relationship of the foreign body with hypertrophic vessel of right bronchial artery. At bronchoscopy a fragment of lamb bone was found

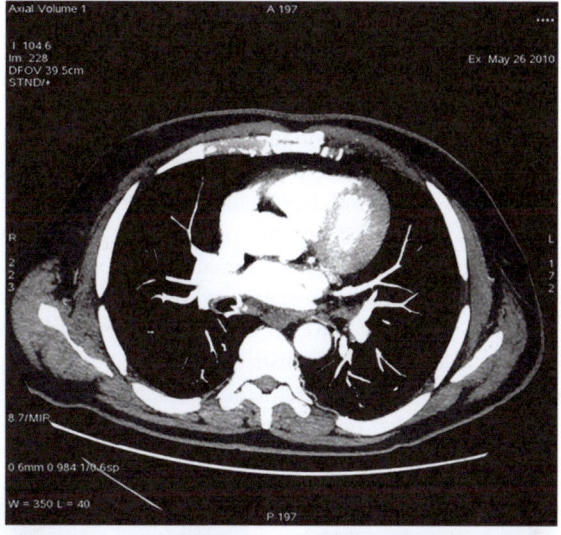

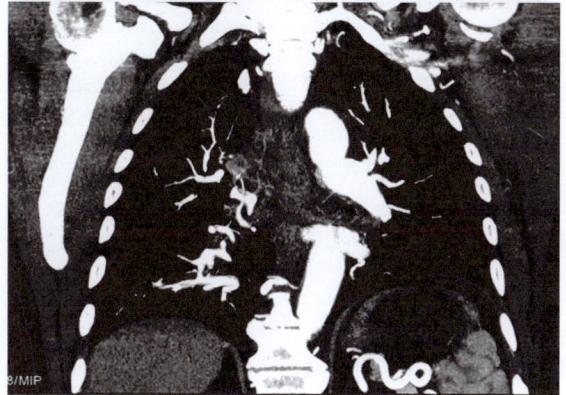

Peculiar: sand or gravel bronchogram

CT signs:

Direct visualization of the foreign body in the tracheo-bronchial tree is best for radiopaque material (Fig. 2.8), [2, 5].

Possibility to visualize radiolucent intrabronchial materials also (Fig. 2.9).

Atelectasis segmental, lobar or of an entire lung.

Obstructive hyperinflation, mediastinal shift.

Obstructive pneumonia.

Air space consolidations with gravitational distribution.

Complications: Localized bronchiectasis, abscess, empyema, emoftoe (Figs. 2.8, 2.12, and 2.13).

Peculiar signs and syndromes:

Alveolar consolidations with perihilar, bilateral, distribution; or patchy infiltrates, segmental or lobar consolidation, usually of the lower lobes, in Mendelson's syndrome.

Centrilobular ill-defined nodules, tree in bud aspect and miliary nodules in granulomatous pneumonitis also called lentil aspiration pneumonia.

Abscess (ill-defined roundend opacities solid or cavitary) in aspiration of infectious material from the oropharynx, especially in patients with poor oral hygiene and advanced periodontal disease.

Signs of pulmonary edema whose gravity depends on the amount of water aspirated (fresh or salt), in near-drowning syndrome: perihilar opacities in subsegmental or segmental distribution with peripheral sparing.

Air–space opacities that tend to coalesce throughout both the lungs.

Sand or gravel bronchogram in near-drowing or motor vehicle collisions.

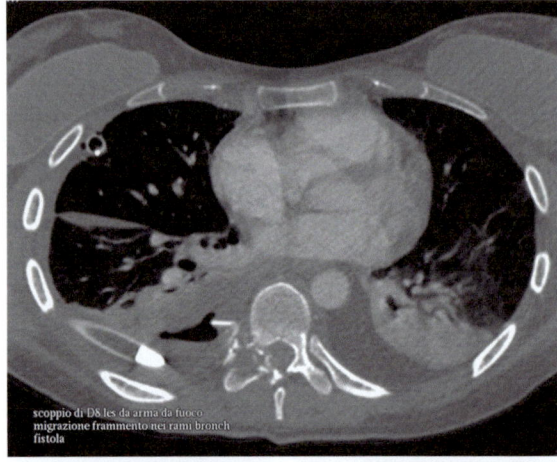

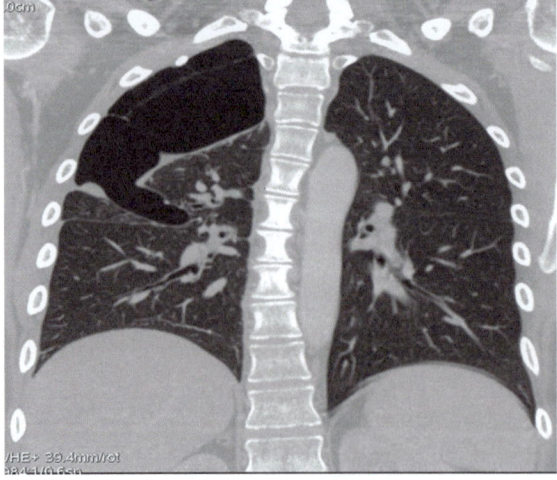

Fig. 2.14 A challenging case: sharper traumatic foreign body, not aspirated, in a segmental bronchus of right lower lobe. Burst lesion of D8 in a polytrauma patient with migration of fragment in the bronchial tree and creation of bronchopleural fistula and pneumothorax

Fig. 2.15 3D visualization of stenosis of medial third of the trachea

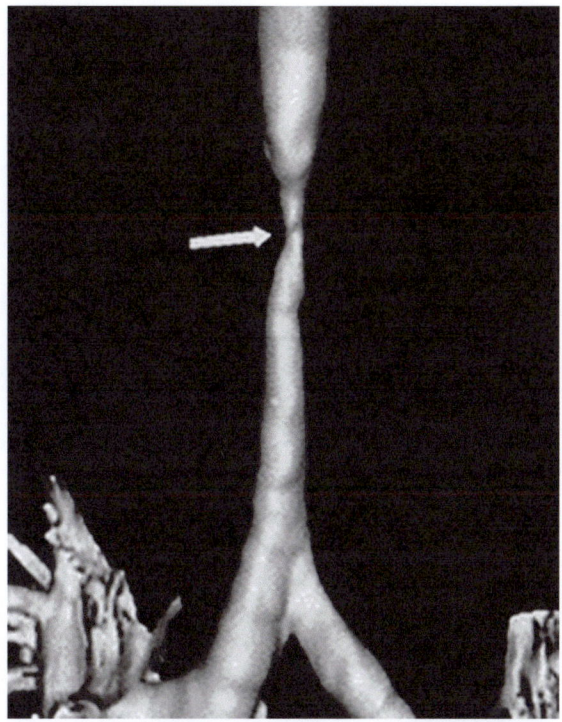

Areas of consolidation characterized by fat attenuation or crazy paving in exogenous lipoid pneumonia.

Confluent opacities in aspiration of hydrocarbure (Fig. 2.10) nodules; and pneumatoceles in fire-eater pneumonia.

Chest devices as tubes and stents positioned in the tracheobronchial-tree may be considered foreign bodies: they can induce foreign body reactions and complications.

Endotracheal tube is a device required for mechanical ventilator; when correctly positioned the tip of the tube should be located several centimeters above the tracheal carina (5 cm in the patient in the neutral position), to allow excursions of 2 cm requested by neck movement of extension or flexion. Malpositioned endotracheal tube most commonly enters the right main bronchus determining atelectasis of the left lung and hyperinflation of the right and eventually pneumothorax. A tip located too high at the level of hypopharynx or larynx may determine poor ventilation or gastric distension; if at the level of the vocal cords tube's tip can cause ulceration and scarring with stenosis.

Malpositioned tube can be located also in the esophagus and is associated with gastric distension and unusual position of the tube in the lateral view. [6].

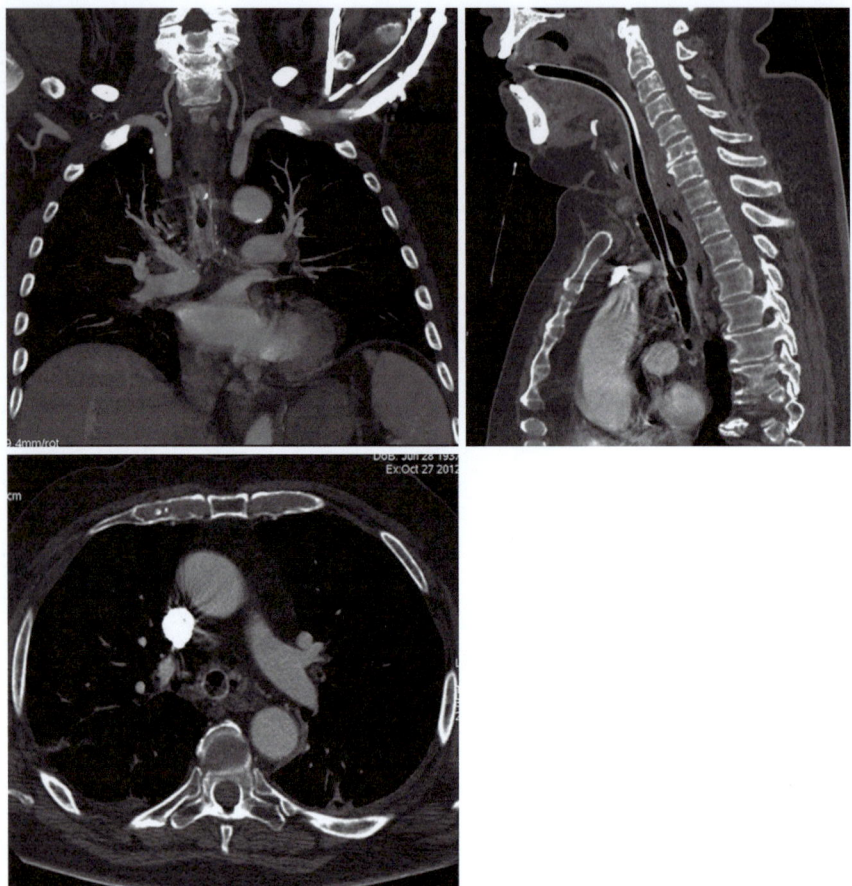

Fig. 2.16 Dislocated Dumon prosthesis with lower margin at the carena and orotracheal tube

Overinflation of the tube cuff or balloon results in compression of the vessels of the anterolateral tracheal wall with ischemic alteration leading to malacia and stenosis [7, 8].

Tracheostomy tube is required for chronic mechanical ventilation or in case of upper airway obstruction. Prolonged intubation may complicate with stenosis at the site of the tracheostomy stoma, at the end of the tube (in the point of contact of the tip with the tracheal mucosa) or more frequently at the level of the inflatable cuffed balloon (usually 1.5 cm below the stoma). The inflated balloon compresses the mucosa against the tracheal rings determining ischemia and erosion of the tracheal wall with subsequent perforation and cicatricial stenosis.

Critical stenosis is characterized by a lumen less than 5 mm, with inspiratory dyspnea at rest, stridor, and triage.

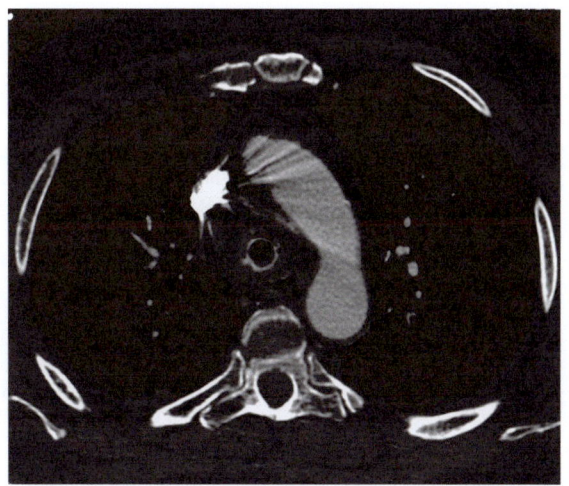

Fig. 2.17 Inflammatory circumferential thickening of tracheal wall in close relationship with the lower margin of the dislocated prosthesis

The stenosis may by fixed (involving both inspiratory and expiratory phase) or variable (only inspiratory or expiratory).

Tracheal or tracheobronchial stents are more frequently used to treat obstructions due to either benign or malignant processes. The type most frequently used to treat benign stenosis (mainly post intubation) is actually the Dumon stent, entirely made of silicon, because it is easier to remove. Nitinol stents are indicated for neoplastic stenosis (Figs. 2.14, 2.15, 2.16, and 17).

Complications are related to stent migration (Fig. 2.15), recurrence of stenosis due to tissue hyperplasia, stent fracture, and difficulty of stent removal.

Bronchial stents are occasionally used in transplanted lung for anastomotic stenosis between the native tracheobronchial tree and the transplanted one.

MDCT provides non-invasive, excellent visualization of the airways due to the possibility to generate multiplanar reformations, MiniP, 3D volume rendered images, and virtual bronchoscopy [9–11].

It allows the careful visualization of the airways, the type of the stenosis (location of the stenosis, precise extent, and the morphologic characteristics (abrupt transition or tapered transition)), the direct visualization of the stents, and the related complication.

References

1. Tomás Franquet MD, Ana Giménez MD, Nuria Rosón MD, SofíaTorrubia MD, José M. Sabaté MD, Carmen Pérez MD (2000) Aspiration diseases: findings, pitfalls, and differential diagnosis. Radiographics 20:673–685
2. Zissin R, Shapiro-Feinberg M, Rozenman J, Apter S, Smorjik J, Hertz M (2001) CT findings of the chest in adults with aspirated foreign bodies. Eur Radiol 11:606–611

3. Farhad Baharloo MD, Francis Veyckemans MD, Charles Francis MD, FCCP, Marie-Paule Biettlot RN, Daniel O, Rodenstein MD (1999) Tracheobronchial foreign bodies presentation and management in children and adults. Chest 115:1357–1362
4. Marom E, McAdams HP, Erasmus JJ, Goodman PC (1999) The many faces of pulmonary aspiration. AJR 172:121–128
5. Zagalo C, Santiago Æ N, Grande ÆNR, Martins dos Santos J, Brito ÆJ, Aguas ÆAP (2002) Morphology of trachea in benign human tracheal stenosis: a clinicopathological study of 20 patients undergoing surgery. Surg Radiol Anat (2002) 24:160–168
6. Kim JH, Shin JH, Song H-Y, Shim TS, Yoon CJ, Ko G-Y (2007) Benign 9 tracheobronchial strictures: long-term results and factors affecting airway patency after temporary stent placement. AJR 188:1033–1038
7. Karen M. Horton, Maureen R. Horton, Elliot K. Fishman (2007) Advanced visualization of airways with 64-MDCT: 3D mapping and virtual bronchoscopy.AJR 189:1387–1396
8. Kosucu P, Ahmetoglu A, Koramaz I et al (2004) Lowdose MDCT and virtual bronchoscopy in pediatric patients with foreign body aspiration. AJR 183:1771–1777
9. Honnef D, Wildberger JE, Das M, Hohl C, Mahnken AH, Barker M, Günther RW, Staatz G (2006) Value of virtual tracheobronchoscopy and bronchography from 16-slice multidetector-row spiral computed tomography for assessment of suspected tracheobronchial stenosis in children. Eur Radiol 16:1684–1691
10. Kim M, Lee KY, Lee KW, Bae KT (2008) MDCT Evaluation of foreign bodies and liquid aspiration pneumonia in adults. AJR 190:907–915
11. Tim B, Hunter MD, Mihra S, Taljanovic MD, Pei H, Tsau MD, William G, Berger MD, James R, Standen MD (2004) Medical devices of the chest. Radiographics 24:1725–1746
12. Taha MS, Mostafa BE, Fahmy M, GhaVar MKA, Ghany EA (2009) Spiral CT virtual bronchoscopy with multiplanar reformatting in the evaluation of post-intubation tracheal stenosis: comparison between endoscopic, radiological and surgical findings. Eur Arch Otorhinolaryngol 266:863–866

Foreign Bodies of the Gastrointestinal Tract

Antonio Pinto, Silvana Nicotra and Vincenzo Di Mauro

3.1 Introduction

Cases of a foreign body (FB) in the gastrointestinal (GI) tract are not common, but are important. These may be caused by accidental ingestion, iatrogenic related, or voluntarily ingested or inserted for personal satisfaction [1]. Most swallowed FBs are not problematic because they pass through the GI tract and are excreted naturally. However, some FBs may result in severe complications, such as bowel obstruction or perforation, hemorrhage, abscess formation, and/or septicemia [1]. In the United States, 1,500 people die each year due to ingested foreign bodies [2].

The diagnosis of an ingested or inserted foreign body is often overlooked in those patients who cannot report an adequate history. Key factors influencing patient management include the type of object, its physical characteristics, the location of the object, the time elapsed since its ingestion, associated medical conditions, the presence or absence of symptoms, and evidence of complications.

The first diagnostic tool for the evaluation of patients with suspected gastrointestinal tract FBs is radiography. Multidetector row Computed Tomography (MDCT) is rarely needed to diagnose FBs, but occasionally it is used to detect ingested objects that are missed by other modalities. MDCT is also helpful in the

A. Pinto (✉) · S. Nicotra
Department of Diagnostic Radiological Imaging, Cardarelli Hospital,
Via Cardarelli 9, 80131 Naples, Italy
e-mail: antopin1968@libero.it

S. Nicotra
e-mail: silvananicotra@hotmail.it

V. D. Mauro
Department of Biomorphological and Functional Sciences, University Federico II of Naples,
Via Pansini 5, 80131, Naples, Italy
e-mail: vin.dimauro@alice.it

detection of FB complications, such as perforation, fistula, or abscess [3]. It is important to remember that failure to demonstrate a FB radiographically does not preclude its presence.

The GI tract can be divided into several regions in which presentation, clinical findings, and management of FBs is distinct. These regions include the oropharynx, esophagus, stomach and duodenum, small and large intestine, and rectum. In this chapter the relevant imaging features for impacted FBs in each of these regions are presented.

Oropharyngeal Foreign Bodies

Most ingested FBs do not become impacted in the oropharynx. The most common exceptions are fish or chicken bones (Fig. 3.1), although any sharp or irregular object may become impacted [4]. These objects most often lodge in the soft tissue at the base of the tongue, but may also be found in other areas such as the tonsil or piriform sinus [4]. Patients usually know exactly when the object became impacted. Typically they present to the Emergency Department (ED) with a FB

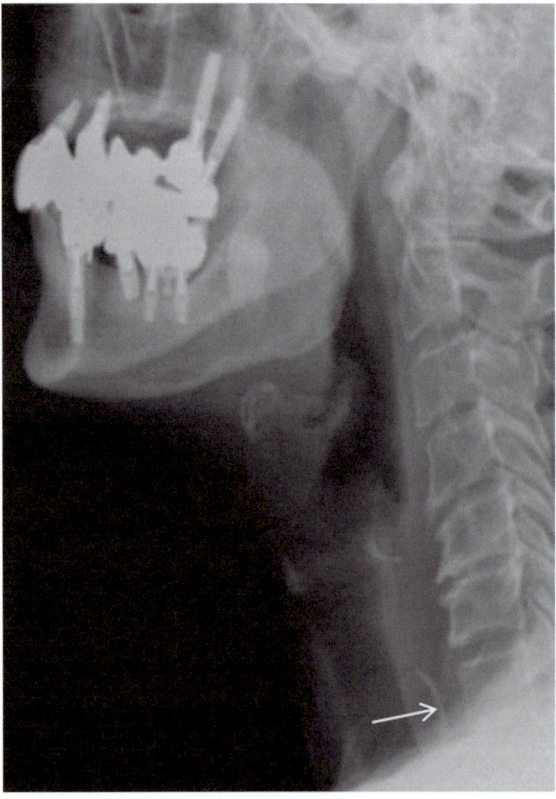

Fig. 3.1 Lateral plain film shows the presence of a radiopaque foreign body (chicken bone) (*arrow*) anterior to the body of C7

sensation and odynophagia several hours after ingestion, and they may have attempted one or more home remedies such as drinking fluid, eating bread, or trying to grasp the object with their own fingers [5]. Hypopharyngeal foreign bodies can be detected with a good physical examination and an indirect laryngoscope examination. However, as related in Western countries [6] most of the FBs are located in cervical esophagus, where they cannot be detected, and then the otolaryngologist must search for additional information from endoscopy or radiology [6]. The radiological visualization of a FB depends on its radiopacity [7]. FBs in the esophagus are much more likely to be radiopaque. Coins are the most commonly impacted object in children. Food products are the second most common and can be confirmed on plain films when spicules of bone or cartilage are present. Perforation of the pharyngeal or esophageal wall is possible [8], and migration of the FB in the adjacent tissues can be facilitated by swallowing, coughing, and esophageal peristalsis [9], as well as by the weakening of the pharyngeal wall due to the local inflammation [10]. Recently, MDCT imaging has been found useful for the evaluation of patients with suspected pharyngoesophageal FBs because it offers short examination time and the ability to obtain diagnostically useful coronal and sagittal reconstruction images. MDCT can detect ingested objects such as slightly calcified objects that are missed by conventional radiographs. Moreover, MDCT is also helpful to detect FB complications, such as perforation, fistula, or abscess [11].

Esophageal Foreign Bodies

The esophagus is another common site for impaction of FBs that are accidentally or purposefully swallowed. Patients who have esophageal FBs can be loosely classified into four groups: (1) pediatric patients, (2) psychiatric patients and prisoners, (3) patients who have underlying esophageal disease, and (4) edentulous adults. The largest group is the pediatric group, which corresponds to 75–80 % of cases. Most of these children are aged 18–48 months [12]. Anatomic features of the esophagus are important to identify because there are areas that are at risk of FB impaction. The first area is located posterior to the cricoid cartilage, at the level of the C6 vertebra, where the esophagus begins with the upper esophageal "sphincter" or cricopharyngeus muscle. The second is at the level of T4 where the distal aortic arch descends posterior to the midesophagus [5]. Distally, there is also an area of narrowing at the lower esophageal sphincter (LES). The LES is the narrowest point of the entire gastrointestinal tract in adults, and it is the location where most FBs become impacted [13]. Many materials can lodge in the esophagus; they can be classified as food bolus impactions or true FBs. True FBs can be subdivided into blunt objects, sharp objects, and miscellaneous (narcotic packs and disk batteries). The most commonly encountered upper esophageal FBs include dental work, coins (Fig. 3.2), bones, and fruit pits. Other frequently encountered objects in children include crayons, marbles, small toys, keys, stones, and safety

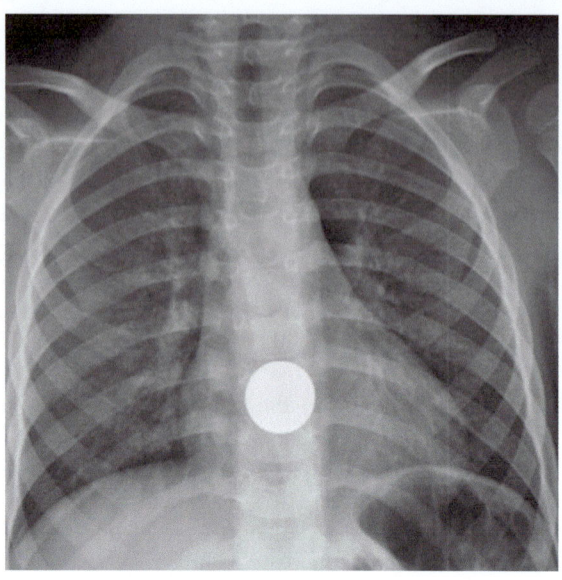

Fig. 3.2 Chest radiograph shows the presence of a radiopaque foreign body (coin) lodged at the level of the distal portion of the thoracic esophagus

pins. FBs are common causes of noniatrogenic esophageal injury. Complications from perforation of the hypopharynx and upper esophagus include retropharyngeal abscess [14], mediastinitis, and even rare instances of aortoesophageal fistulas or tracheoesophageal fistula [15, 16], penetration of the common carotid [17] and facial artery [18], thyroid abscess [19], and epidural abscess [20]. The first diagnostic tool for the evaluation of patients with suspected pharyngoesophageal FBs is radiography. Many objects, such as meat, tiny bones, aluminum, glass, plastic, and wood, may be radiolucent and not visualized on plain radiographs [21]. Although some of these objects may be detected when oral contrast is given, there is a limited role for contrast studies in the management of FBs. Barium studies should be avoided if there is clinical evidence of high-grade obstruction or there is suspicion of esophageal perforation, as there is the potential for barium spillage into the mediastinum or pleural space. If barium is used, a minimal amount of a thin solution is preferred, as residual barium in the esophagus obscures visualization during a subsequent endoscopy. Gastrografin may be helpful in localizing a suspected perforation, but because of its hypertonicity, it may cause severe pneumonitis if aspirated [21].

Stomach and Duodenal Foreign Bodies

The vast majority of FBs that enter the stomach pass through the entire GI tract uneventfully. Objects longer than 5 cm may have difficulty negotiating the tight curve of the duodenum, and objects larger than 2 cm in diameter may have difficulty passing the pylorus or ileocecal valve [22, 23]. Less than 1 % of FBs that enter the stomach cause perforation of the bowel [24].

Battery ingestions (Fig. 3.3) are common among children, impaired individuals, and those with psychiatric disorders. There are four types of button batteries that range in size from 6 to 23 cm: manganese dioxide, silver oxide, mercuric oxide, and lithium manganese. The larger the diameter of the battery, the more likely it is to lodge in the esophagus. The possible mechanisms of injury from battery ingestion include leakage of battery contents, electrical discharge, and pressure necrosis. Another potential mechanism of injury is absorption of heavy metals from broken or fragmented batteries. However, no cases of heavy metal poisoning from disc battery ingestion have been reported. The alkaline solutions in these batteries can cause liquefaction necrosis and saponification in the mucosal surface of the GI tract. If the battery remains in place, ulceration and perforation can occur.

Foreign Bodies of the Small and Large Intestine

Once in the small intestine, the most common impaction point is the ileocecal valve, followed by the hepatic and splenic flexures. Less than 1 % of ingested foreign bodies cause perforation of the gastrointestinal tract. Sharp, elongated objects (Fig. 3.4) are the most likely to penetrate the bowel mucosal lining and cause significant injury to the bowel wall or frank perforation [1].

Two interesting phenomena occur that help protect the bowel wall from injury during foreign body passage. The first is related to axial flow and a tendency for sharp objects to be turned in the intestine so that the sharper end will trail down the lumen. Second, once the foreign object reaches the colon, it becomes surrounded by fecal material that aid in bowel wall protection.

Management of sharp FBs in the intestine includes daily radiographs to document progression of the FB. If there is no distal progression over a 3-day period

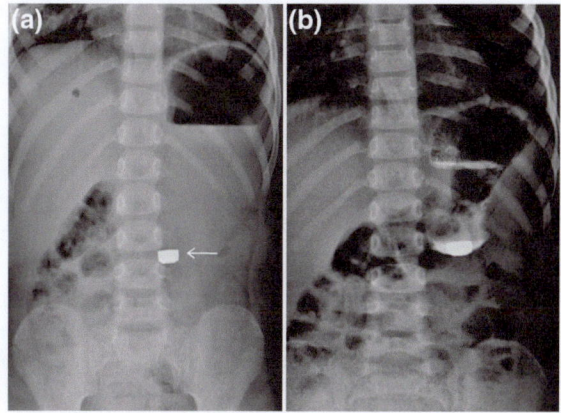

Fig. 3.3 Plain abdominal film shows an ingested radiopaque foreign body (battery) (**a**, *arrow*). The exact location of the ingested foreign body is confirmed after oral administration of gastrografin (**b**)

Fig. 3.4 Plain abdominal film shows an ingested radiopaque foreign body (nail) (*arrow*) located at the level of the distal portion of the descending colon

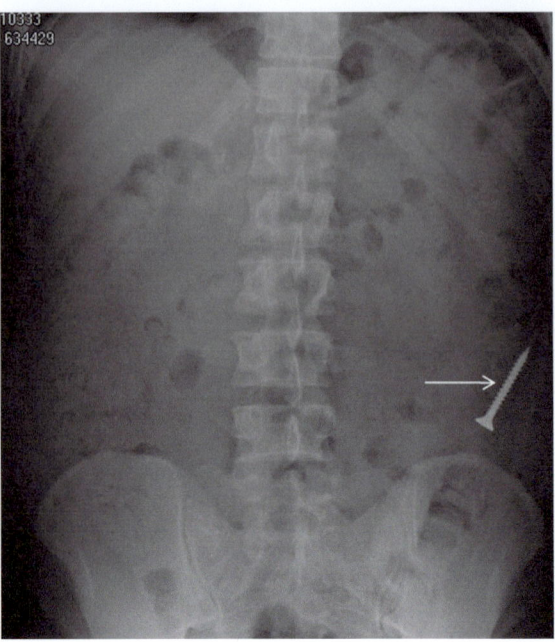

or if the patient becomes symptomatic, emergent surgical consultation should be obtained [25].

MDCT is regarded to be a good modality for detecting and characterizing FBs in the GI tract and for evaluating the risk of complications. However, metallic FBs produce beam-hardening artifacts, which can obscure their contours and those of surrounding structures. Although scout MDCT images can be helpful for identifying FBs, they have lower resolution than plain radiographs. The majority of FB ingestion patients essentially need close observation and monitoring by serial plain radiography. Furthermore, because MDCT has a greater radiation hazard than plain radiography, plain radiography is the better alternative for follow-up examinations particularly in the paediatric population.

Rectal Foreign Bodies

The number of patients presenting with retained rectal foreign bodies appears to have increased in recent decades. Foreign objects retained in the rectum may result from ingestion or direct introduction through the anus (more common). Affected individuals often will make unsuccessful attempts to remove the object themselves, resulting in further delay of medical care and potentially increasing the risk of complications. As with upper GI foreign bodies, the types of objects introduced through the anus are unlimited. Objects such as vibrators, rubber phallus, vegetables (carrots, zucchini, corn cob) (Fig. 3.5), fruit (apple, banana), stones, wire,

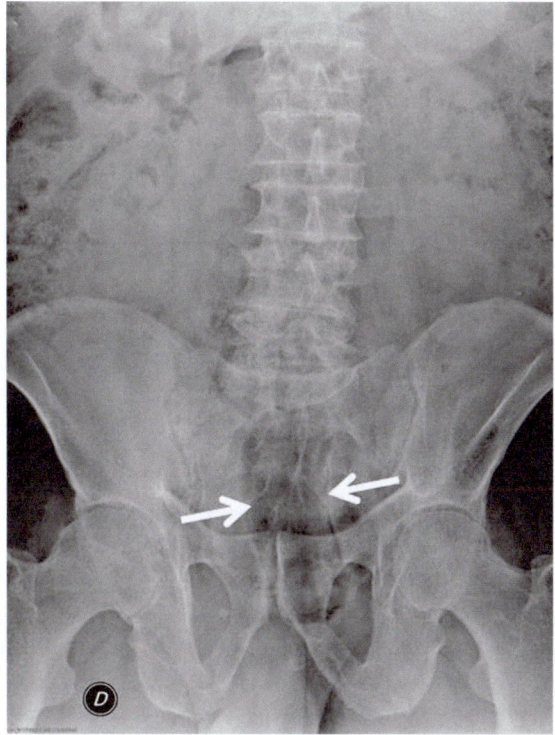

Fig. 3.5 Plain abdominal film shows a radiolucent foreign body (vegetable) (*arrows*) located at the level of the rectum

toothbrush, screwdrivers, rodents, cans, bottles, and jars are but a few of the retained rectal objects reported. Autoeroticism has been reported as the most common reason for anally inserted foreign bodies [26]. Diagnostic problems can occur with trans-anal rectal injuries, because of the natural hesitancy of the patient to describe what might have been a very embarrassing and socially unacceptable incident. Trans-anal high hydrostatic pressure may cause severe colorectal injury, necessitating resection of the blown injured segment. The firm lateral support of the rectum makes the rectosigmoid junction the first part to be hit by the pressure column, which acts as a solid body as it opens the anal sphincter [3].

Body Packing

Over the last two decades, drug smuggling has not only increased worldwide, but the gastrointestinal tract has been also used more frequently as a vehicle for smuggling narcotics [27, 28]. Body packing and body stuffing are the terms employed for intracorporeal concealment of illicit drugs, mainly cocaine and heroine. The general characteristics of a body packer include: (1) returning from a trip abroad in a location with a history of illicit drug exporting; (2) history of frequent trips; (3) high profit drugs such as cocaine or heroin involved; and (4) the packaging material is made of high-grade latex, aluminum foil, or condoms. In addition to transporting cocaine and heroin, body packers may smuggle amphetamines, 3,4-methylenedioxymethamphetamine ("ecstasy"), marijuana, or hashish. Occasionally, they ingest more than one type of drug. Body packers usually carry about 1 kg of drug, divided into 50–100 packets of 8–10 g each, although persons carrying more than 200 packets have been described [28]. Patients suspected of being body packers require radiographic evaluation. Plain abdominal X-ray is the most widely used radiological tool to detect drug-filled packets of 2–8 cm within the gastrointestinal tract of body packers [27, 29, 30]. However, due to limited contrast resolution, conventional radiographs (CR) of body packers reveal the presence of drug containers in 40–90 % of cases only [27, 28, 31–33]. Several specific signs on the abdominal radiograph may suggest the presence of body packing: multiple radiodense foreign bodies, a "rosette-like finding" formed by air trapped in the knot where a condom is tied [27, 32] and a "double-condom" sign [27, 31] in which air trapped between layers of latex makes them more visible. The last finding may also suggest a loss of integrity of the packing material [34]. Abdominal ultrasound (US) [27] and radiographic studies after oral intestinal opacification with hydrosoluble contrast agents have been used and recommended for investigation of body packers. However, for detection of the small-sized cocaine-filled packets, which may be located anywhere in the digestive tract, none of these two methods is considered very sensitive [30].

Magnetic resonance imaging (MRI) is rarely used as first-line emergency modality, because of high costs and limited availability. The best imaging modality for revealing foreign bodies is Multi-detector row Computed Tomography (Fig. 3.6), which is superior to abdominal radiographs and ultrasound in terms of sensitivity, localization, and characterization of density [35]. Schmidt et al. [36] reported the good diagnostic value of unenhanced CT for the detection of cocaine-filled packets. Their radiological appearance is based on the presence of an air–solid interface: an outer halo of air, provided by the wrapped cellophane

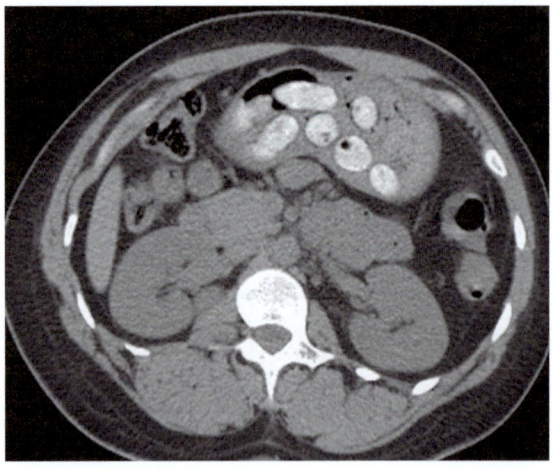

Fig. 3.6 Unenhanced abdominal MDCT scan showing multiple hyperdense foreign bodies located in the stomach

containing tiny amounts of air trapped during the packing surrounding the central cocaine [36]. This so-called "double-condom" sign is considered the key feature of drug-filled condoms of body packers on plain films [27, 29, 33] and on CT [37].

Cocaine-filled packets appear as focal high-density areas on CT [31]. Eng et al. reported one case of false negative CT of the abdomen without contrast in a

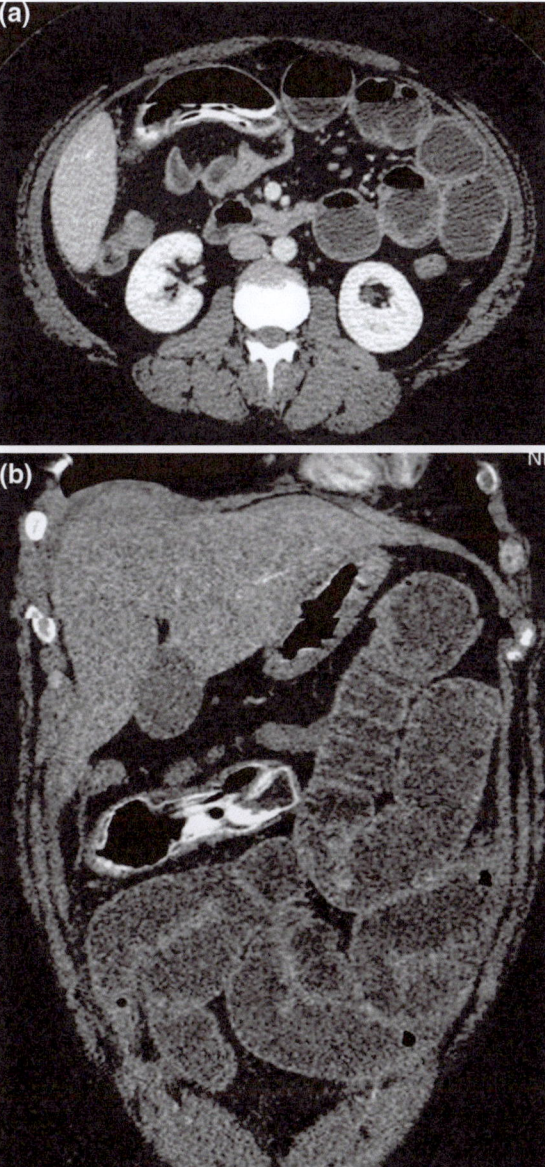

Fig. 3.7 Enhanced abdominal MDCT (**a**, axial scan and **b**, coronal scan) showing a small bowel obstruction due to migration of an esophageal stent

cocaine body stuffer [38]. Moreover, Sengupta et al. [39] recommend the simple step of reviewing CT scans of suspected body packers on altered windowing and standard abdominal windowing to improve the detection of fatty drug packages.

Bowel obstruction is commonly reported in body packers; the level of obstruction is usually at the ileocecal valve; the urgency in impacted cocaine-filled condoms is due to the risk of transmucous absorption and its potentially lethal consequences. Bowel wall perforation, peritonitis, esophageal obstruction, and esophageal perforation are less frequently noted [28]. Radiologists should be aware that bowel obstruction with all consecutive complications may be caused by foreign bodies. Careful reading of plain X-ray films of the abdomen and a high skill in doing ultrasound is needed not to miss the underlying cause of an acute abdomen. If there exists any suspicion of drug packets in the intestine, MDCT may be used as a further diagnostic tool [40].

Foreign Bodies from Prior Surgical Procedures

Stents and endoprostheses are used with increasing frequency in malignant and refractory benign stenoses of the biliary and gastrointestinal tract. Stents used to overcome malignant biliary and gastrointestinal stenoses are made of plastic or metal. Stents to treat the latter, usually made of nitinol or stainless steel, can be bare, partially covered (at the center), or covered [41].

Stents may be deployed incorrectly or may dislodge after a variable interval of time after placement. Migration seems to occur more frequently with covered stents, probably because of their weaker anchorage, than with uncovered stents [41]. Although usually spontaneous, stent migration may sometimes be caused by surgical, endoscopic, or percutaneous maneuvers [42]. Stent migration may cause obstruction (Fig. 3.7), hemorrhage, and perforation [43] or may have no consequence. The checklist for radiologists interpreting images showing stents includes determining stent type, purpose, position, patency, and integrity and identifying persistent tissue (inflammation, free air, fluid or contrast material, enhancement, bleeding) if present.

3.2 Conclusions

A wide variety of FBs may be encountered by plain radiography, which is the primary imaging modality used to evaluate patients with an FB in the GI tract. The diagnosis and the management of patients who have ingested or inserted FBs depends on a number of factors, such as the anatomic location of the FB, the kind and size of the FB.

In patient with an ingested or inserted foreign body, the goals of the initial patient assessment are to determine the type of object, its location in the gastrointestinal tract, the presence of any associated complications, and the presence of any underlying gastrointestinal conditions.

References

1. Hunter TB, Taljanovic MS (2003) Foreign bodies. Radiographics 23:731–757
2. Schwartz GF, Polsky HS (1976) Ingested foreign bodies of the gastrointestinal tract. Am Surg 42:236–238
3. Pinto A, Sparano A, Cinque T (2012) Foreign body ingestion and rectal foreign body insertion: diagnostic challenges. In: Romano L, Pinto A (eds) Errors in radiology, Springer Italia, pp 271–278
4. Wu I, Ho T, Chang C et al (2008) Value of lateral neck radiography for ingested foreign bodies using the likelihood ratio. J Otolaryngol Head Neck Surg 37:292–296
5. Anderson KL, Dean AJ (2011) Foreign bodies in the gastrointestinal tract and anorectal emergencies. Emerg Med Clin N Am 29:369–400
6. Marco De Lucas E, Sádaba P, Lastra Garcıa-Barón P et al (2004) Value of helical computed tomography in the management of upper esophageal foreign bodies. Acta Radiol 45:369–374
7. Pinto A, Scaglione M, Pinto F et al (2006) Tracheobronchial aspiration of foreign bodies: Current indications for emergency plain chest radiography. Radiol Med 111:497–506
8. Pinto A, Muzj C, Stavolo C et al (2004) Pictorial essay: Foreign body of the gastrointestinal tract in emergency radiology. Radiol Med 107:145–154
9. Cheng YC, Lee WC, Kuo LC et al (2009) Protrusion of a migrated fish bone in the neck. Am J Otolaryngol 30:203–205
10. Kanne JP, Mann FA (2004) Pharyngeal perforation from an impacted fish. AJR Am J Roentgenol 182:802
11. Pinto A, Muzj C, Gagliardi N et al (2012) Role of imaging in the assessment of impacted foreign bodies in the hypopharynx and cervical esophagus. Semin Ultrasound CT MRI 33:463–470
12. Stack LB, Munter DW (1996) Foreign bodies in the gastrointestinal tract. Emerg Med Clin North Am 14:493–521
13. Conway WC, Sugawa C, Ono H et al (2007) Upper GI foreign body: An adult urban emergency hospital experience. Surg Endosc 21:455–460
14. Poluri A, Singh B, Sperling N et al (2000) Retropharyngeal abscess secondary to penetrating foreign bodies. J Craniomaxillofac Surg 28:243–246
15. Scher RL, Tegtmeyer CJ, McLean WC (1990) Vascular injury following foreign body perforation of the esophagus. Review of the literature and report of a case. Ann Otol Rhinol Laryngol 99:698–702
16. Loh KS, Tan LK, Smith JD et al (2000) Complications of foreign bodies in the esophagus. Otolaryngol Head Neck Surg 123:613–616
17. Osinubi OA, Osiname AI, Pal A et al (1996) Foreign body in the throat migrating through the common carotid artery. J Laryngol Otol 110:793–795
18. Chung SM, Kim HS, Park EH (2008) Migrating pharyngeal foreign bodies: A series of four cases of saw-toothed fish bones. Eur Arch Otorhinolaryngol 265:1125–1129
19. Lu PK, Brett RH, Aw CY et al (2000) Migrating oesophageal foreign body—An unusual case. Singapore Med J 41:77–79
20. Tsai YS, Lui CC (1997) Retropharyngeal and epidural abscess from a swallowed fish bone. Am J Emerg Med 15:381–382
21. Smith MT, Wong RK (2007) Foreign bodies. Gastrointest Endosc Clin N Am 17:361–382

22. Knight LC, Lesser TH (1989) Fish bones in the throat. Arch Emerg Med 6:13–16
23. Koch H (1977) Operative endoscopy. Gastrointest Endosc 24:65–68
24. Johnson WE (1969) On ingestion of razor blades. JAMA 208:2163
25. Webb WA (1995) Management of foreign bodies of the upper gastrointestinal tract: update. Gastrointest Endosc 41:39–51
26. Cohen JS, Sackier JM (1996) Management of colorectal foreign bodies. J R Coll Surg Edinb 41:312–315
27. Hierholzer J, Cordes M, Tantow H et al (1995) Drug smuggling by ingested cocaine-filled packages: conventional x-ray and ultrasound. Abdom Imaging 20:333–338
28. Traub SJ, Hoffman RS, Nelson LS (2003) Body packing–the internal concealment of illicit drugs. N Engl J Med 349:2519–2526
29. Pinsky MF, Ducas J, Ruggere MD (1978) Narcotic smuggling: the double condom sign. J Can Assoc Radiol 29:79–81
30. Hergan K, Kofler K, Oser W (2004) Drug smuggling by body packing: what radiologists should know about it. Eur Radiol 14:736–742
31. Pollack CV Jr, Biggers DW, Carlton FB Jr et al (1992) Two crack cocaine body stuffers. Ann Emerg Med 21:1370–1380
32. Beerman R, Nunez D Jr, Wetli CV (1986) Radiographic evaluation of the cocaine smuggler. Gastrointest Radiol 11:351–354
33. Sporer KA, Firestone J (1997) Clinical course of crack cocaine body stuffers. Ann Emerg Med 29:596–601
34. McCleave NR (1993) Drug smuggling by bodypackers: detection and removal of internally concealed drugs. Med J Aust 159:750–754
35. Gor DM, Kirsch CF, Leen J et al (2001) Radiologic differentiation of intraocular glass: evaluation of imaging techniques, glass types, size, and effect of intraocular hemorrhage. AJR Am J Roentgenol 177:1199–1203
36. Schmidt S, Hugli O, Rizzo E et al (2008) Detection of ingested cocaine-filled packets– Diagnostic value of unenhanced CT. Eur J Radiol 67:133–138
37. Meyers MA (1995) The inside dope: cocaine, condoms, and computed tomography. Abdom Imaging 20:339–340
38. Eng JG, Aks SE, Waldron R et al (1999) False-negative abdominal CT scan in a cocaine body stuffer. Am J Emerg Med 17:702–704
39. Sengupta A, Page P (2008) Window manipulation in diagnosis of body packing using computed tomography. Emerg Radiol 15:203–205
40. Pinto A, Stavolo C, Muzj C (2012) Radiological and medico-legal problems of body-packing. In: Romano L, Pinto A (eds) Errors in radiology, Springer, Italia, pp 279–286
41. Catalano O, De Bellis M, Sandomenico F et al (2012) Complications of biliary and gastrointestinal stents: MDCT of the cancer patient. AJR Am J Roentgenol 199:W187–W196
42. Brinkley M, Wible BC, Hong K et al (2009) Colonic perforation by a percutaneously displaced biliary stent: report of a case and a review of current practice. J Vasc Interv Radiol 20:680–683
43. Görich J, Rilinger N, Krämer S et al (1997) Displaced metallic biliary stents: technique and rationale for interventional radiologic retrieval. AJR Am J Roentgenol 169:1529–1533

Intra-Abdominal Foreign Bodies: Gossypiboma and Abdominal Wall Meshes

Nicola Gagliardi, Nicoletta Pignatelli Di Spinazzola, Vincenzo Di Mauro, Giuseppe Ruggiero and Carlo Muzj

4.1 Introduction

Intra-abdominal foreign bodies, in most cases, consist of surgical sponges, because a gauze soaked with blood and packed in some abdominal recess can easily get out of control and visibility. Indeed, unintentional retention of a surgical sponge inside the human body during surgery is a serious event and highly feared by every surgeon.

Although the possibility of "forgetting" a sponge during surgery is unacceptable, no other surgical treatise has dedicated an important chapter to this well-known and widely reported topic in their series [1].

This event is, above all, a big problem for the patient and is one of the issues most frequently reported in medical malpractice that strongly impresses the public. It is a source of great fury to lawyers and leads to great severity of judgment by Judges in the court of law [2].

It is estimated that this complication can intervene at least once in every 5,000 operations, but the estimation is difficult particularly due to the low susceptibility to spontaneous reporting of the event [3].

Surgical sponges are also referred to as gossipybomas. This term is derived from the Latin word *gossypium*, meaning cotton, and the Swahili word *boma*, meaning place of concealment. Recently, with the increasing use of synthetic sponges, as retained objects they are referred to as textiloma [3, 4].

N. Gagliardi (✉) · N. Pignatelli Di Spinazzola · G. Ruggiero · C. Muzj
Department of Diagnostic Radiological Imaging, CT Body Unit, Cardarelli Hospital,
Via A. Cardarelli, 9 – 80131, Naples, Italy
e-mail: n.gagliardi@katamail.com

V. Di Mauro
Department of Diagnostic Imaging and Radiotherapy, Federico II University, Naples, Italy

The incidence does not seem related to the experience of the surgeon or the surgical team, but rather to the most experienced surgeons, because performing complex interventions could lead to this complication.

Situations of surgical sponge forgetfulness in the abdomen include: surgical procedures performed in emergency, duration and complexity of the intervention, unexpected complication as hemorrhage, unexpected changes and then unplanned procedures during surgery, obesity of patient, interventions that involve more than one surgical team, situations that favor the counting error as gauzes stuck together or defective packages [2, 5].

In most countries, surgical sponges contain radio-opaque marking filaments that facilitate their detection by standard abdominal radiography and on computed tomography (CT) images. Older sponges do not always include radio-opaque markers and therefore they can be very difficult to identify on standard radiography and CT [6]. Delayed diagnosis of gossypibomas could increase mortality and morbidity.

Abdominal wall repairing meshes, in some cases, may act as foreign bodies, more frequently when complications occur. Indeed, since some meshes are radio-opaque (PTFE meshes), if the mesh is detached from the abdominal wall it can generate a radiographic image very similar to gossipyboma, especially if a seroma or an abscess is present [7].

This is especially true in incisional hernia repair using large meshes and when, as a result of inflammation, calcium gets deposited on the mesh.

Metal fixation stitches on the abdominal wall, if present, and the medical history of patient can help in diagnosis [8].

4.2 Complications

The complications that gossipyboma may determine are extremely variable and depend on the site and elapsed time. A surgical sponge can be encapsulated by a fibrotic reaction and give few symptoms, either absent or present with a bowel obstruction from fibrotic adhesions or pseudotumoral syndrome. It may result in an abscess with infection and sepsis symptoms or can migrate inside of hollow organs (bowel, bladder) resulting in perforation and damage to the concerned organs [9, 10].

Because retained sponges can mimic tumor both clinically and radiologically, and their manifestations and complications are so variable, diagnosis is difficult and often delayed and patient morbidity is significant. Gossipyboma may become symptomatic at any time and usually necessitates reoperation for removing the gauze and for the treatment of complications. Mortality is important as the range between 11 and 35 % in different series [11].

Abdominal wall meshes, if displaced, lead to problems of differential diagnosis with gossipyboma. The factors that generate mesh displacement are insufficient size, incorrect placement, defective material, immediate displacement by folding, lifting by a hematoma, late displacement by insufficient scar tissue growth, mesh protrusion, collagen disease, or pronounced shrinkage [12]. If an abdominal mesh is displaced or prolapsed and an inflammatory reaction in present, it can simulate a foreign body in abdominal cavity due to adhesions to the peritoneum.

Also, in this case the symptoms are variable and can appear after a long time, and the clinical diagnosis is often difficult [13].

4.3 Radiologic Findings

The diagnosis of intra-abdominal foreign bodies is based on many characteristic radiologic findings for gossipyboma and for displaced abdominal wall meshes.

This diagnosis is often difficult because these findings may be unusual and dissimilar.

Consequently, and given the legal implications of this diagnosis, particularly for gossipyboma, it is essential that the radiologist is familiar with and is able to detect everyone necessary for a proper diagnosis. What is required is precise diagnosis which can supply the clinician with any necessary information for a proper therapeutic decision [14].

Standard Radiography

Planar abdominal radiography is the first diagnostic step to detect foreign bodies. In case of sponges, if there is a radio-opaque marker, detection and diagnosis can be made quite easily. Conversely, if the sponge is radiolucent, diagnosis may be very difficult (Fig. 4.1). In some cases standard abdominal radiography is a fine opacity area as a soft-tissue mass characterized by small gas bubbles in and around structure [14]. However, this technique cannot determine the relationship between the sponge and the abdominal structures. The diagnosis is easier when a whirl-like pattern of radio-opaque thread is seen on the radiography, but unfortunately this finding is not always present (Fig. 4.2) [4, 14].

The advantage of this technique, in suspected sponge forgetting in abdominal cavity, is related to the possibility to perform the investigation immediately after surgery with a portable X-ray machine, when the patient is still in the operating theater under anesthesia.

If gossipyboma has resulted in fistula formation, oral contrast may be administrated to help in its identification and thus the correct diagnosis [15].

Displaced abdominal wall meshes is a rare event, linked to the occurrence of complications after surgery. In most cases, only the staples that fix the mesh to the abdominal fascia are seen with plain abdominal radiography (Fig. 4.3) [7].

Usually indeed, the mesh is translucent and does not appear visible. In addition, this technique does not show accurately the presence of complications.

Fig. 4.1 Gossipyboma: radiolucent material (surgical drape) is seen on *left side* (*arrowheads*)

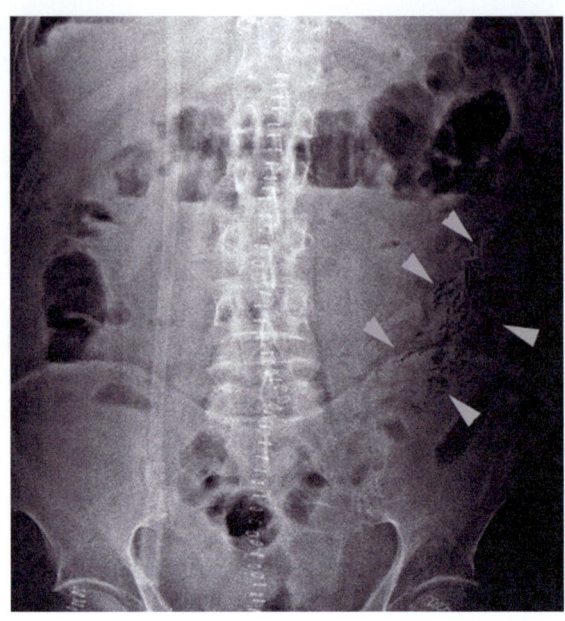

Fig. 4.2 Gossipyboma: radiolucent material (*arrowhead*) and radio-opaque marker (*arrow*) are seen on *upper left side* after splenectomy

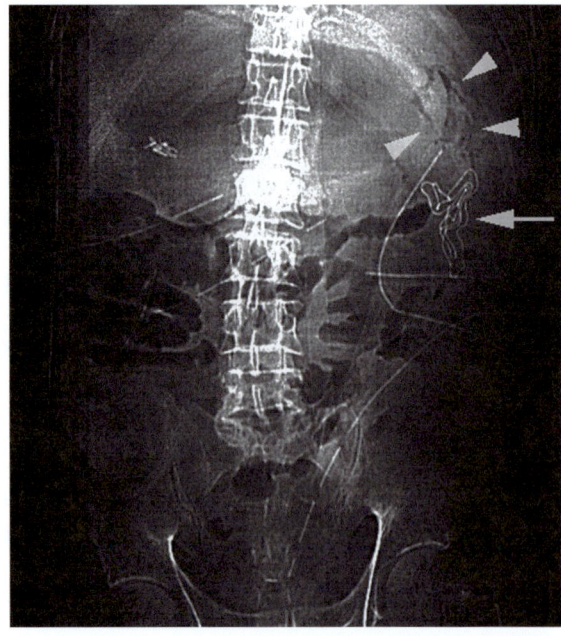

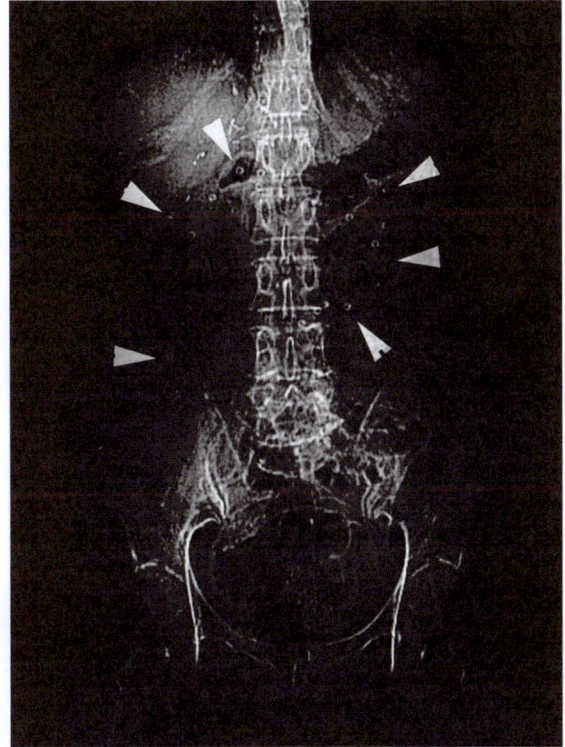

Fig. 4.3 Plain abdominal radiograph in a patient with incisional hernia repair. Only the staples (*arrowhead*) that fix the mesh to the abdominal fascia are seen with this technique

US

A surgical sponge retained in the abdominal cavity can often be detected sonographically. Its characteristic appearance is a well-delineated and hyper-reflective lesion with wavy internal echo, strong posterior shadow, and hypoecoic ring [16]. At ultrasound images we recognize sponges as cystic or solid type mass. The former consist of a cystic lesion with a winding echogenic bundle, and the latter as a complex structured mass with hyper and hypoechoic areas (Fig. 4.4) [17].

The pattern of acoustic shadowing changes with the direction of the ultrasound beam but is caused by material itself, indicating calcified regions or a pocket of air. The sonographic detection of a mass with high echoes casting acoustic shadows should alert radiologists to the likelihood of retained surgical sponges.

Abdominal wall meshes on ultrasound appear as hyperechoic lines. Sonographically, we can identify postoperative complication as fluid collection and we can differentiate between hematoma or seroma (Fig. 4.5). In some cases, especially those in which septa or air is noted inside the collection, it is difficult to make the distinction.

Also, purulent collection around the mesh and bowel complication due to adhesion or mesh displacement is identified by ultrasound easily [17].

Displacement only without complications is not identifiable by ultrasound.

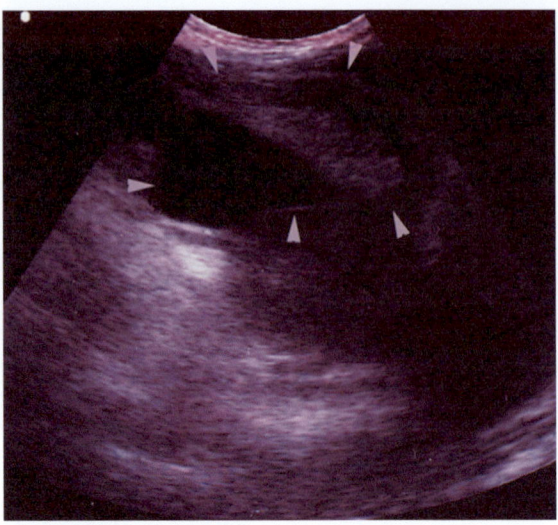

Fig. 4.4 An abdominal mass of complex structure (gossipyboma) adherent to the anterior peritoneum

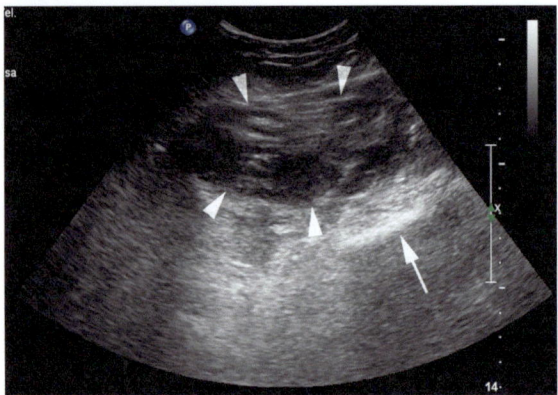

Fig. 4.5 Abdominal wall e-PTFE mesh seen as hyperechoic lines (*arrow*) displaced by hematoma (*arrowheads*)

CT

Gossipyboma and their possible complications are best identified on CT. Most authors describe well-circumscribed disomogeneus masses with a thick wall, often with gas bubbles inside, sometimes without showing calcification or wall enhancement after administration of i.v. contrast medium (Fig. 4.6a, b) [14]. The internal structure of such masses may be whirl-like or spongiform due to gas-trapped bubbles in the sponge. It may be of low density or complex, with both low density and wavy, striped or spotted high-density areas (Fig. 4.7) [18]. The radio-opaque marker strip is of a thin metallic density in the mass (Fig. 4.8a, b).

Spongiform pattern with gas bubbles inside is the most specific CT sign for the presence of gossipyboma, but sometimes a long-lasting sponge will resemble a

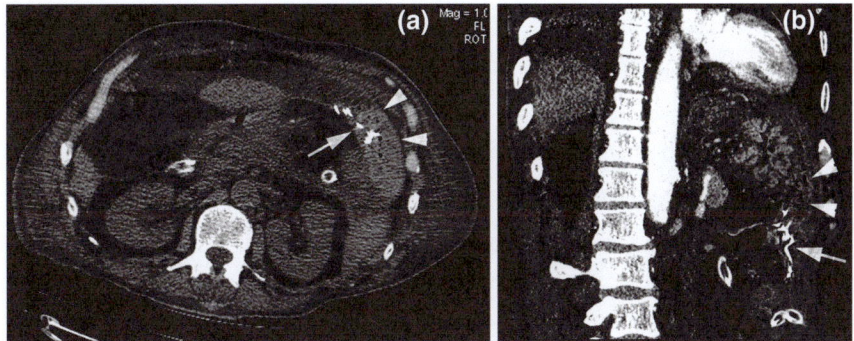

Fig. 4.6 The same case as in Fig. 4.2a, b Gossipyboma in *upper left side*, with a spongiform pattern (*arrowheads*) and radio-opaque marker (*arrows*)

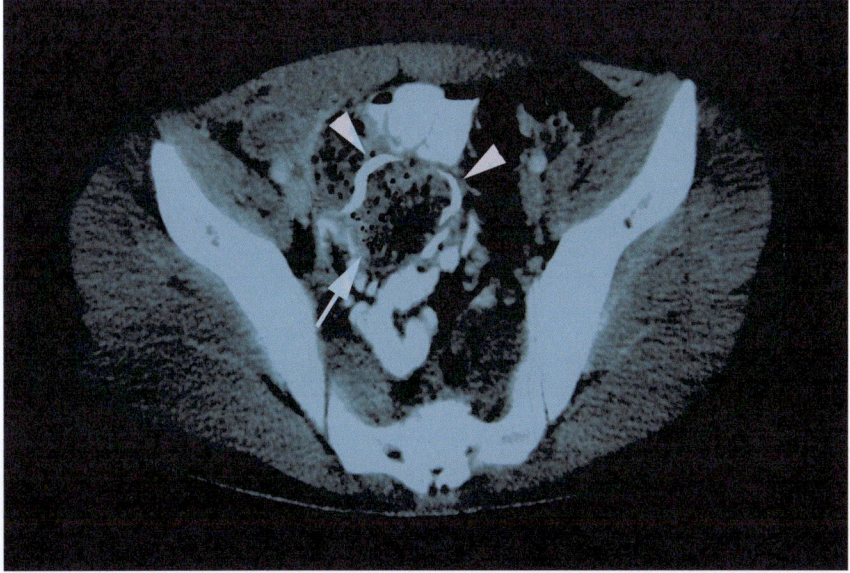

Fig. 4.7 Gossipyboma in the right iliac fossa after hemicolectomy, with radio-opaque marker (*arrowheads*) and spongiform pattern (*arrow*)

cystic mass bounded by a calcified ring (Fig. 4.9a, b). The reticulated and calcified appearance of the internal portion of the mass is due to the gradual calcification along the fibers of the surgical gauze [19]. Diagnostic misinterpretation is due to variable appearance of gossipyboma. This pitfall sometimes results in unnecessary surgical procedures.

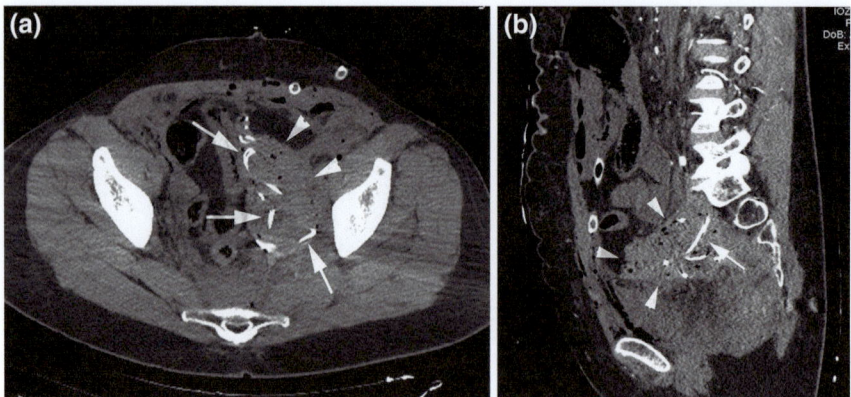

Fig. 4.8 Gossipyboma in left iliac fossa after small bowel resection. **a,b** Solid mass with air bubbles inside (*arrowheads*) and radio-opaque marker (*arrows*)

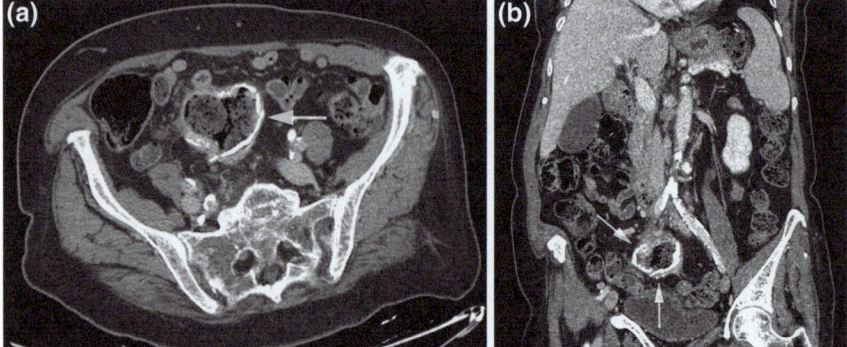

Fig. 4.9 Gossipyboma in hypogastric area. **a, b** Inhomogeneous mass with similar-fecal material inside and radio-opaque marker around (*arrows*)

The appearance of abdominal wall meshes on CT, likely because of their different composition and thickness, is different from polypropylene (PP) meshes and expanded-polytetralfluorethylene (e-PTFE) meshes. The PP meshes are visible as lines with density similar to the adjacent muscles in only a small proportion of patients (Fig. 4.10). The e-PTFE meshes appear as a line of increased density visible in all patients [7, 20].

Their twisted appearance and the presence of complications such as hematoma and seroma indicate a displacement, especially if they are distant from the fastening staples (Fig. 4.11).

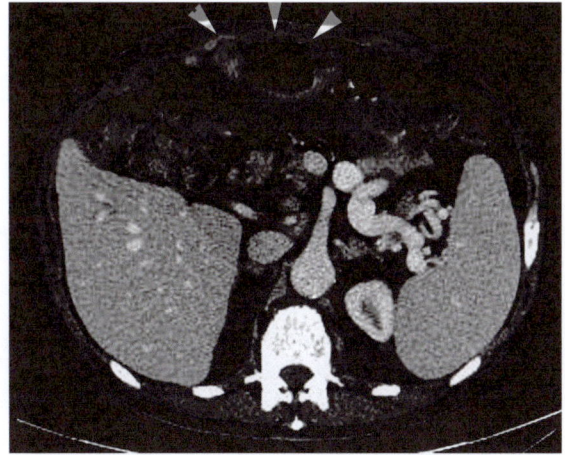

Fig. 4.10 PP abdominal with bowel adhesion after inflammatory complication. The PP mesh appears as a line with density similar to the adjacent muscles (*arrowheads*)

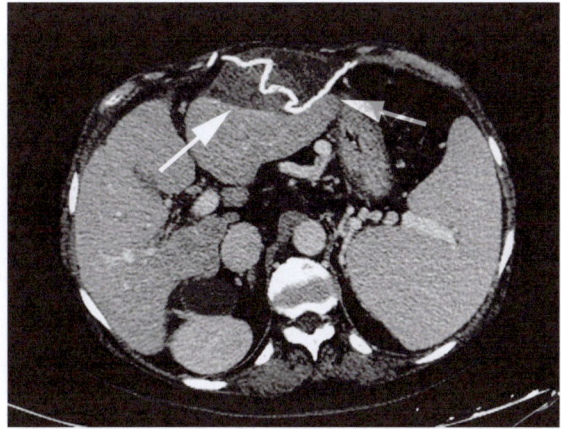

Fig. 4.11 Displaced abdominal wall e-PTFE mesh in lenticular hematoma of anterior abdominal wall (*arrows*)

MRI

To date, only a few reports on the MRI appearance of gossypiboma in the abdomen and pelvis have been published. On MRI, the signal intensity of the mass will vary according to its histologic composition, stage, and fluid content. A retained surgical sponge is typically seen as a soft-tissue density mass with a thick well-defined capsule; on T2-weighted imaging it has a whorled internal configuration [21].

References

1. Stawicki SP, Evans DC, Cipolla J et al (2009) Retained surgical foreign bodies: a comprehensive review of risks and preventive strategies. Scand J Surg 98:8–17
2. Shyung LR, Chang WH, Lin SC et al (2005) Report of gossipyboma from the standpoint in medicine and law. World J Gastroenterol 11:1248–1249
3. Kernagis LY, Siegelman ES, Torigian DA (2009) Case 145: retained sponge. Radiology 251:2
4. Manzella A, Borba Filho P, Albuquerque E et al (2009) Imaging of gossypibomas: pictorial review. AJR 193:S94–S101
5. Sun HS, Chen SL, Kuo CC et al (2007) Gossipyboma-retained surgical sponge. J Chin Med Assoc 70(11):511–513
6. Tzu-Chieh Cheng, Andy Shau-Bin Chou, Chin-Ming Jeng et al (2007) Computed tomography findings of gossypiboma. J Chin Med Assoc 70:565–569
7. Parra JA, Revuelta S, Gallego T et al (2004) Prosthetic mesh used for inguinal and ventral hernia repair: normal appearance and complications in ultrasound and CT. B J Radiol 77:261–265
8. Crovella F, Bartone G, Fei L (2008) Incisional hernia. Springer ,Italia
9. Gencosmanoglu R, Inceoglu R (2003) An unusual cause of small bowel obsctruction: gossypiboma—case report. BMC Surg 3:6
10. Haegeman S, Maleux G, Heye S et al (2008) Texiloma camplicated by abscess formation, three years after surgical repair of abdominal aortic aneurysm. JBR-BTR 91:51–53
11. Kaiser CW, Friedman S, Spurling KP et al (1996) The retained surgical sponge. Ann Surg 224:79–84
12. Flament JB, Avisse C.,Palot JP et al Complications in incisional hernia repairs by the placement of retromuscular prostheses. Hernia 4:S25–S29
13. Leber GE, Garb JL, Alexander AI et al Long-term complications associated with prosthetic repair if incisional hernia. Arch Surg 133:378–382
14. O'Connor AR, Coakley FV, Meng MV et al (2003) Imaging of retained surgical sponges in the abdomen and pelvis. AJR 180:481–489
15. Parasad S, Krishnan A, Limidi J et al (1999) Imaging features of gossypiboma: report of two cases. JPGM 45:18–19
16. Jain M, Jain R, Sawhney S (1995) Gossypiboma: ultrasound-guided removal. J Clin Ultrasound 23:321–323
17. Ersoy H, Saygili OB, Yildirim T (2004) Abdominal gossypiboma: ultrasonography and computerized tomography findings. Turk J Gastroenterol 15(1):65–66
18. Cheng TC, Chou ASB, Jeng CM et al (2007) Computed tomography findings of gossypiboma. J Chin Med Assoc 70:565–569
19. Lu YY, Cheung YC, Ko SF et al (2005) Calcified reticulate ring sign: a characteristic feature of gossypiboma on computed tomography. World J Gastroenterol 11:4927–4929
20. Lin BH, Vargish T, Dachman AH (1999) CT findings after laparoscopic repair of ventral hernia. AJR Am J Roentgenol 172:389–392
21. Kim CK, Park BK, Ha H (2007) Gossypiboma in abdomen and pelvis: MRI findings in four patients. AJR 189:814–817

Abdominal Compartment Syndrome Due to Hepatic Packing

Ciro Acampora, Ciro Stavolo and Maria Paola Belfiore

5.1 Introduction

Damage control surgery is defined as a rapid termination of an operation after control of life-threatening bleeding and contamination followed by correction of physiologic abnormalities and definitive management [1]. Most damage control procedures are performed in the abdomen. This specific technique used is dependent on the nature of the injury. The most common abdominal injuries that induce a damage control approach are liver injuries and abdomen vascular injuries. Damage control is applied when the initial laparotomy is ended and expeditious indirect methods are applied to control massive bleeding or soiling or both [2]. The primary method of hemorrhage control for complex liver injuries is packing.

5.2 Packing

Packing is a result of improvements in surgical management to control the hemorrhage and high associated morbidity from rebleeding and intra-abdominal sepsis. Problems related to packing technique are "overpacking" and "underpacking." "Underpacking" occurs when the packing is inadequately performed and the consequence is the immediate failure due to ongoing hemorrhage. Likewise, when it is excessively performed as "overpacking," it may lead to multiorgan failure (MOF) or abdominal compartment syndrome (ACS) [3]. ACS is caused by packs

C. Acampora (✉) · C. Stavolo
Department of Diagnostic Radiological Imaging, Cardarelli Hospital,
Via Cardarelli 9, Naples, Italy
e-mail: itrasente@libero.it

M. P. Belfiore
Second University of Naples (SUN), Piazza Miraglia 2, Naples, Italy

fixed between the abdominal wall and hepatic parenchyma with consequent traction of the hepatic and inferior cava veins. Thus, it is indicated and a decision is made to perform packing; it should be done in order by placing the proper number of packs in the right locations [4]. The criteria for inadequate packing include hemodynamic instability, low hematocrit values, even after the transfusion of many units of blood, insertion of an intra-abdominal drainage catheter, and signs of inappropriate packing procedure (the number of packs fewer than required or packs placed in wrong locations) in the re-look operation. The most common problem with this technique is the determination of timing for the placement and removal of the packs and the method that should be used. The decision to pack should be made early in the exploration in order to provide better chance of survival for liver trauma patients [5]. Patients with uncontrollable bleeding caused by pelvic fractures are also eligible for packing [6]. The patients with active hemorrhage from the drain placed in the first operation and persistent hemodynamic instability were submitted to an early operation. If there was enough time, considering the patient's hemodynamic criteria, routine computed tomography was also done to determine the extent of the injury. It is mainly used in the presence of a lesion major liver and to a lesser extent in lesions retroperitoneal and pelvic.

Damage control surgery for liver injury consists of a midline laparotomy with minimal liver mobilization and an initial four-quadrant packing to investigate any additional intra-abdominal injury. Ongoing bleeding from the liver led to liver packing. Failure to control bleeding led to packing the liver systematically with 5–8 abdominal packs, considering the capacity of the intra-abdominal cavity, in order to restore liver continuity and to obtain right compression. Temporary closure techniques were applied if there were any concerns about intra-abdominal pressure. Perihepatic packing procedure, which is the basic control technique to arrest hepatic hemorrhage, is one of the cornerstones of trauma surgery and, currently, this is the most commonly accepted and performed method for major liver trauma [3]. The main goal after packing is to correct acidosis, hypothermia, and coagulopathy, the lethal triad causing death. Packing is performed using laparotomy pads placed with a goal to compress the source of hemorrhage. The goal is tamponade bleeding while maintaining organ perfusion. Complications following packing procedures may be due to bleeding, especially in "underpacking" cases or to MOF syndrome, in "overpacking" to excessive intra-abdominal pressure to allow ACS [5].

5.3 Abdominal Compartment Syndrome

The compartment syndrome is a condition of increased pressure in a confined anatomic space that adversely affects the circulation and threatens the function and viability of the tissues therein. This may arise in any closed compartment within the body [6]. ACS is characterized by increased intra-abdominal pressure associated with organ dysfunction. In primary ACS, the cause is a disease or injury of an abdominal organ, while in secondary ACS the cause is outside the abdomen.

The normal intra-abdominal pressure is about 5 mmHg in critical patient (physiological pressure change occurs with the breaths, coughing, defecation, and Valsalva maneuver). In ACS, the intra-abdominal pressure reaches a value of around 20 mmHg with dysfunction in at least one chest-abdominal organ [7–11]. The high mortality of this complication makes necessary early identification since in most cases the decompression laparotomy determines an improvement in organ dysfunction [12]. ACS generally occurs in patients with surgical condition as trauma, burns, liver transplantation, retroperitoneal condition, such as ruptured abdominal aortic aneurysm and pancreatitis, and in case of "underpacking" and "overpacking." The diagnosis is mainly clinical and rapidly made by measuring intra-bladder pressure, obtained with a Foley catheter at bedside [7]. In the past, the radiologist's role has been minimal in the definition of the ACS and only in recent years the support of imaging techniques has become essential in certain situations, for example, if it is not possible to perform an examination of the patient in intensive care units, especially in cases where it is not possible to obtain an accurate measurement of intra-bladder pressure, such as neurogenic bladder, packing, or urethral trauma. In addition, patients usually are always subjected to CT examination to measure the severity of underlying disease and to identify any complications, which makes it very useful to identify the early signs of semiotic TC that allow the radiologist to suspect an ACS. Imaging findings that can raise the suspicion of ACS show high sensitivity and low specificity, as the elevation of the diaphragm, the round shape of the CT silhouette in the abdomen, the emo-peri-retroperitoneum, the increased enhancement of the intestinal wall and gastric; while color-Doppler evaluation shows lack of diastolic flow of hepatic artery branches and to and from flow in the portal vein [13]. Pickhardt et al. reported other findings that include collapsed inferior vena cava, tense retroperitoneal infiltration, mass effect on the kidneys, and diffuse bowel-wall thickening [14] (Fig. 5.1). Some of these findings are very early, as the elevation of the diaphragm, because the respiratory symptoms already occur for intra-abdominal pressure around 15 mmHg [15]. However, this radiological sign is not very specific since it can also be present in other disease, as in the intestinal ileus without increase of pressure. In ACS, the rounded appearance of the abdomen is the most useful radiological CT sign, also termed the "round bell sign." The abdomen shape usually is oval, with a predominant transverse diameter than anterior–posterior. The anterior–posterior and transverse diameters are measured in the CT scan, in which the left renal vein crosses the abdominal aorta and connects with the inferior vena cava, without including the subcutaneous fat in the measurement. However this CT sign is present in the case of massive ascites, in which the patient shows no signs of organ failure. Collapsed inferior vena cava and collapsed renal veins are another sign not specific, since they can occur even in the case of hypovolemic shock where the blood pressure is reduced and the intra-abdominal pressure is not high [13]. The increased enhancement of the intestinal mucosa is another initial sign of ACS, because the venous drainage of the intestinal mucosa is early compromised when the intra-abdominal pressure increases. Response to surgical decompression was dramatic

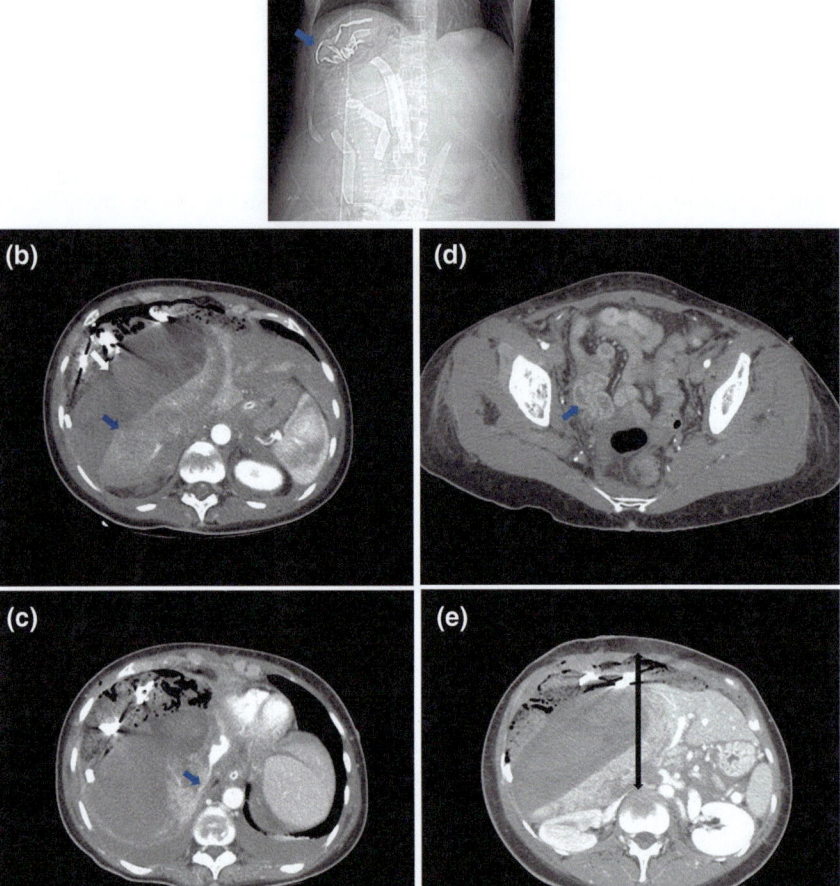

Fig. 5.1 39-year-old woman with ACS as complication of 5° grade liver trauma. Bladder pressure is 35 mmHg measured by Kron method. **a** Scout CT image obtained 4 day after the surgery shows elevated right hemi diaphragm (*white arrow*) and packing (*light blue arrow*). **b** CT image shows big hematoma (*white arrow*) surrounding from "over packing" with hepatic segments lacerations with large ischemia (*light blue arrow*). **c** CT image shows retro hepatic cava vein is over-pressured and clotted (trombizzata) (*light blue arrow*). **d** CT image shows increased enhancement of the intestinal mucosa caused by venous congestion due to hypertension intra-abdominal (*light blue arrow*). **e** CT image shows increased anterior-posterior abdominal diameter studied at level where left renal vein crosses aorta (*black arrow*)

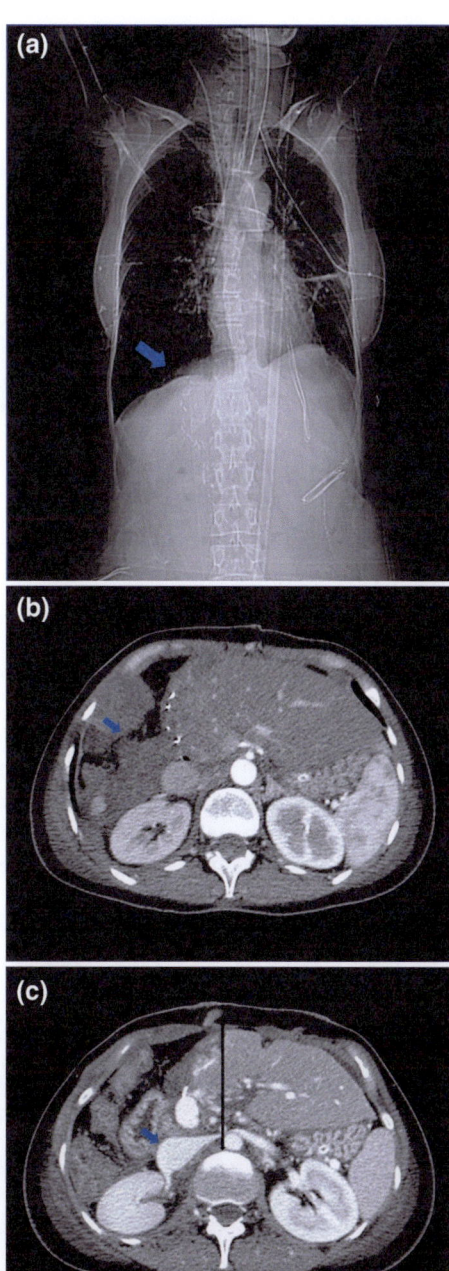

Fig. 5.2 The same patient after decompression surgery. **a** Scout CT image shows normal level of right hemi diaphragm and without packing (*light blue arrow*). **b** CT image shows thin fluid flap along shear section of the right liver (*light blue arrow*). **c** CT image shows the reperfusion of cava and renal veins (*light blue arrow*) and decreased of the anterior-posterior diameter

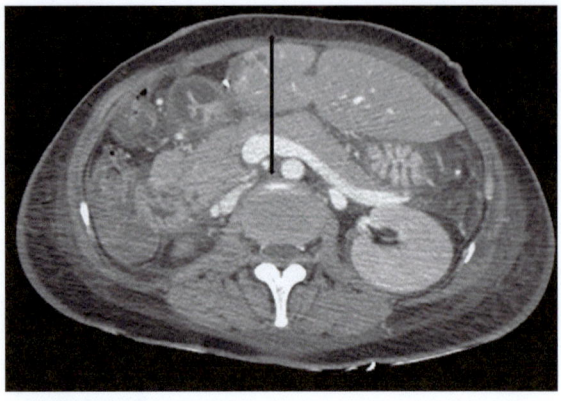

Fig. 5.3 Follow-up after 12 days. CT image shows decreasing of the anterior–posterior diameter with recovering of the ovoid shape

with immediate reversal of organ failure documented by improvement of the pathologic findings, described earlier in the text, at CT imaging (Fig. 5.2).

Follow-up CT scans showed the decompression effect of large open abdominal wound (Fig. 5.3).

Note the recovering of the normal representation of the abdominal structure.

5.4 Conclusion

We can confirm that imaging has a fundamental role in avoiding problems due to incorrect packing procedures, especially to recognize the ACS.

CT is a fundamental method to identify early findings, to help clinics both in diagnosis and therapy. Moreover, diagnostic imaging is very important for follow-up.

References

1. Shapiro MB, Jenkins DH, Schawab W et al (2000) Damage control: collective review. J Trauma 49:969–978
2. Bashir MM, Abu-Zidan FM (2002) Damage control surgery for abdominal trauma. Eur J Surg 588:8–13
3. Aydin U, Yazici P, Zeytunlu M, Coker A (2008) It is more dangerous to perform inadequate packing? World J Emerg Surg 3:1
4. Bach A, Bendix J, Hougaard K, Christensen EF (2008) Resuscitation and emergency medicine. Scand J Trauma 16:4
5. Schreiber M (2004) Damage control surgery. Crit Care Clin 20:101–118
6. Patel A, Lall CG(2007) Abdominal compartment syndrome. AJR 189:1037–1043
7. Kron IL, Harman PK, Nolan SP (1984) The measurement of intra-abdominal pressure as a criterion for abdominal re-exploration. Ann Surg 199:28–30
8. Burch JM, Moore EE (1996) The abdominal compartment syndrome. Surg Clin N Am 76:833–842

9. Ivatury RR, Diebel L (1997) Intra-abdominal compartment syndrome. Surg Clin N Am 77:783–800
10. Tiwari A, Haq AI (2002) Acute compartment syndrome. Br J Surg 89:397–412
11. Meldrum DR, Moore FA (1997) Prospective characterization and selective management of the abdominal compartment syndrome. Am J Surg 174:667–672
12. Chang MC, Miller PR (1998) Effects of abdominal decompression on cardiopulmonary function and visceral perfusion in patients with intra-abdominal hypertension. J Trauma 44(3):440–445
13. Zissin R, Pickhardt PJ (2000) The significance of a positive round belly sign on CT. AJR 175:267–268
14. Pickhardt PJ, Shimony JS (1999) The abdominal compartment syndrome: CT findings. AJR 173:575–579
15. Laffargue G, Taourel P (2002) CT diagnosis of abdominal compartment syndrome. AJR 178:771–772

Foreign Bodies as Complications of Biliary Stents and Gastrointestinal Stents

Antonio Pinto, Daniela Vecchione and Luigia Romano

6.1 Introduction

A stent is a cylindrical medical device used to dilate a narrow or stenosed lumen in order to conserve the patency of the lumen. Currently, stents are increasingly used in blood vessels, in the renal, gastrointestinal, and biliary tracts: In these last anatomical sites, stents (and endoprostheses) are used not only to reestablish patency in malignant and refractory benign stenoses of the biliary and gastrointestinal tract, but also to seal perforations (iatrogenic) and divert flow (fistulas and leaks) [1, 2].

Stents are placed with high success rates (>90 %) [3, 4]. However, complications may develop during positioning, usually being recognized immediately by the operator, or may be discovered after placement by diagnostic imaging, especially by multidetector row computed tomography (MDCT), as early (first 30 days after placement) or late (>30 days) events [2, 5, 6].

Many dislodged tubes may be detected in the gastrointestinal tract, including dislodged feeding tubes and biliary endoprostheses that have migrated from the biliary tract. Most of these objects are related to prior surgery or some other interventional medical procedure. However, a pertinent and complete patient's history is often lacking, since both the patient and the referring physician may be unaware of its relevance for the interpreting radiologist.

A. Pinto (✉) · D. Vecchione · L. Romano
Department of Diagnostic Radiological Imaging, Cardarelli Hospital,
Via A. Cardarelli 9, 80131, Naples, Italy
e-mail: antopin1968@libero.it

D. Vecchione
e-mail: danielavecchione@hotmail.it

L. Romano
e-mail: luigia.romano@fastwebnet.it

The radiologist needs to accurately characterize the exact nature and location of any foreign body that is detected.

6.2 Biliary Stents

Interventional internal drainage of the biliary tract has become an established procedure for both temporary and definitive treatment of biliary obstruction due to malignant or benign disease.

Endoscopic biliary stent placement is a well-established treatment for hepatic, biliary, and pancreatic disorders.

In particular, biliary stents are mostly inserted for the treatment of malignant obstruction caused by pancreatic neoplasm, cholangiocarcinoma, gallbladder cancer, and cancer of the ampulla of Vater. Other indications include biliary fistulae after biliary surgery and patients with bile duct stones where initial attempts at stone extraction are unsuccessful.

Stents may be made of either plastic or metal. Plastic endoprostheses are less expensive but are at higher risk for clogging and dislocation. However, they are frequently used because they are easier to remove or change than metal stents. Most biliary endoprostheses pass through the intestine without any problems.

Complications from stents can develop soon after insertion or can be delayed for weeks or months. Early complications include pain, bleeding, perforation, and stent migration. The most common late complication is stent obstruction because of tumor ingrowth or a food or fecal bolus. The frequency of stent obstruction changes in relation to the type and location of the stent as well as other factors such as diet and use of laxatives. However, the most common cause is ingrowth of tumor. Another complication is stent migration. Distal stent migration (Figs. 6.1, 6.2, 6.3)

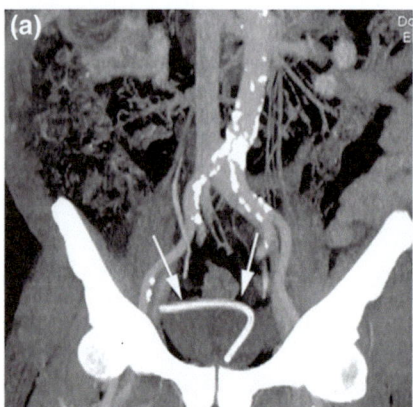
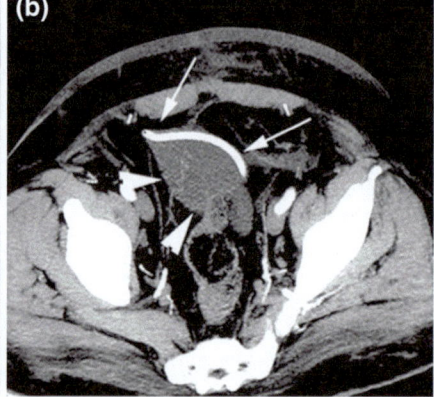

Fig. 6.1 MDCT coronal reformatted image **a** shows a biliary stent (*white arrows*) migrated at the level of the pelvis. MDCT axial image **b** shows a fluid collection (*white arrowheads*) close to the biliary stent (*white arrows*)

Fig. 6.2 Plain abdominal film **a** shows the presence of a biliary stent (*white arrows*): The distal tip of the stent is located in the left paravertebral side. MDCT axial image **b** demonstrates the proximal tip of the biliary stent (*white arrow*) located at the level of the left biliary duct. MDCT axial image **c** reveals the distal tip of the biliary stent (*white arrow*) located into the left mesenteric folds, surrounded by a large fluid collection (*white arrowheads*)

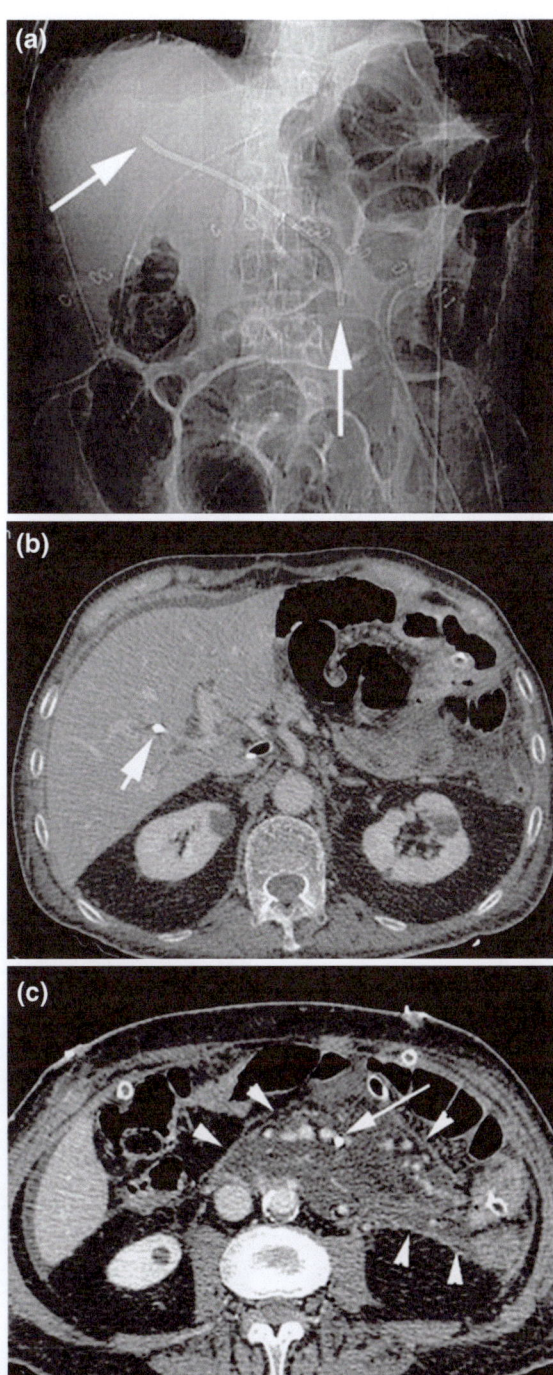

is an uncommon late complication that occurs in up to 6 % of cases [7, 8]: Distal migration may be managed expectantly, allowing the patient to pass the foreign body per rectum [9]. However, when a stent becomes lodged in the intestinal tract, removal is necessary [8]. Complications after stent migration can be classified into

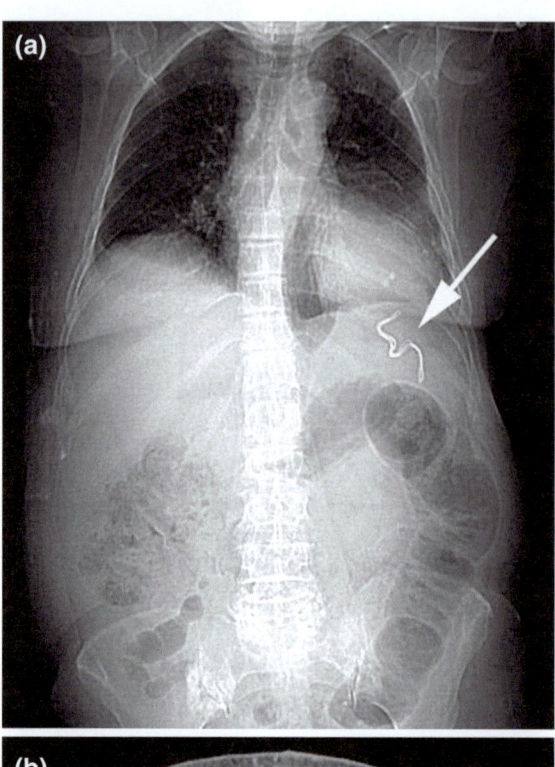
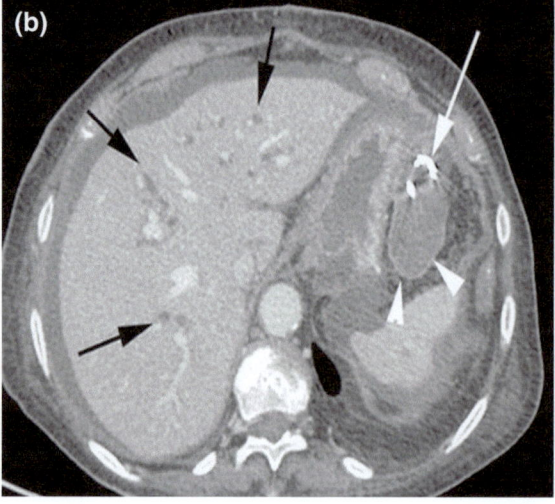

Fig. 6.3 MDCT, scout view **a** a biliary stent fragment (*white arrow*) is located in the left subphrenic space. MDCT, axial image **b** demonstrates the distal pigtail (*white arrow*) of the biliary stent located in the left subphrenic space, surrounded by a fluid collection (*white arrowheads*). The intrahepatic biliary system is enlarged (*black arrows*)

penetration, perforation, and obstruction of the intestine. Rarely, other organs—such as the pleura or pancreas—can be affected [10, 11]. Penetration requires adherence between the perforated organ and another organ. It does not lead to diffuse peritonitis or intra-abdominal contamination, but eventually causes the development of a fistula [12]. Penetration of the intestinal wall can lead to an abscess, which may resolve after stent extraction and conservative treatment [13].

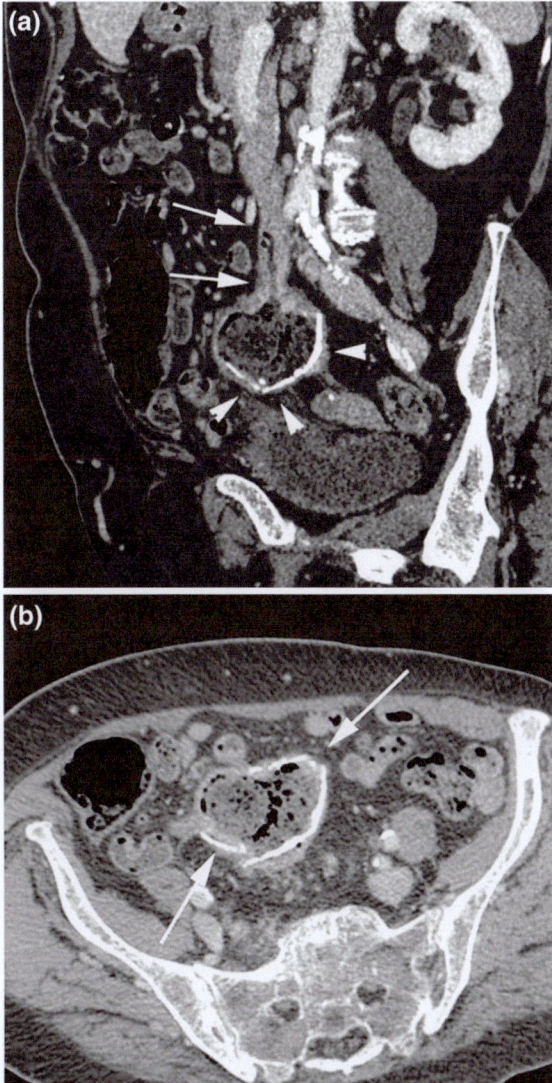

Fig. 6.4 MDCT oblique-coronal reformatted image **a** shows a calcified foreign body (phitobezoar) (*white arrowheads*) thrown out a small bowel loop (*white arrows*). MDCT axial image **b** reveals the calcified foreign body located in the mesenterial folds (*white arrows*)

Known risk factors for distal migration include papillary stenosis, omission of sphincterotomy, use of plastic stents, and stenting of benign lesions. Patients with gastrointestinal symptoms with known stents should be meticulously worked up for the disease requiring stent placement, as well as for the risk of stent migration.

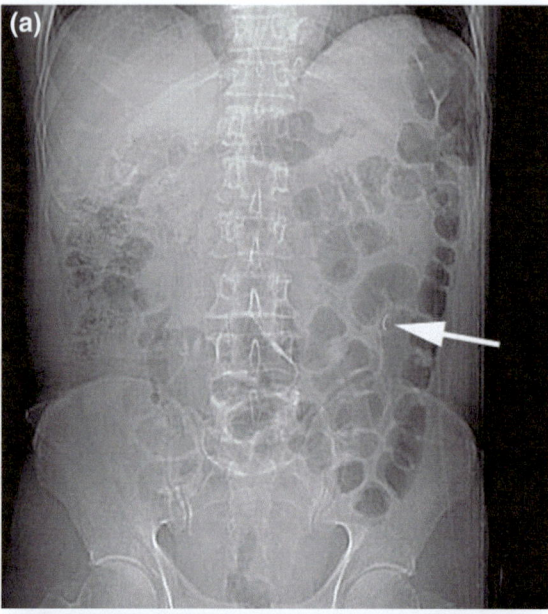
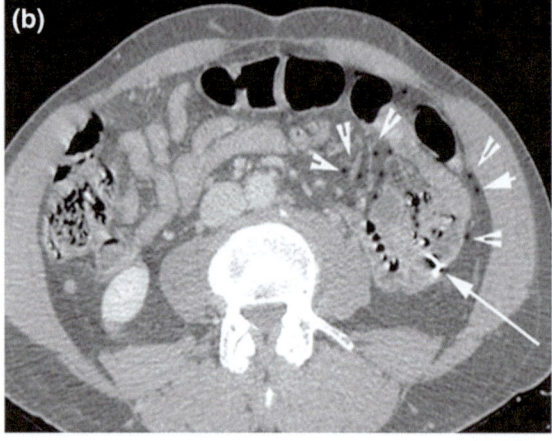

Fig. 6.5 Plain abdominal film **a** shows a metallic foreign body (dental-plate wire) in the lower left abdominal quadrant (*white arrow*). MDCT axial image **b** demonstrates the dental-plate wire blocked in the wall of a small bowel loop (*white arrow*). The loop has been perforated; there are some air bubbles spread in the near mesenterial folds (*white arrowheads*)

6.3 Gastrointestinal Stents

Gastrointestinal stents must be differentiated from other objects that may be found within the lumen of the gastrointestinal tract, as a result of a pathologic condition, e.g., bezoars (Fig. 6.4), swallowing of a diagnostic device (e.g., endoscopic capsules), or accidental or nonaccidental ingestion of some other object (e.g., batteries).

In particular, ingestion of items of odontogenic origin (Fig. 6.5) by patients under general anesthesia or in elderly patients, including dislodged teeth, crowns, fixed partial dentures, and removable partial and complete dentures is not frequent but often goes unnoticed initially, leading to potentially dangerous late complications that require surgical intervention [14].

In the elderly population, especially in patients with dementia, dental prostheses appear to be the most commonly ingested foreign bodies in this population [15]. The main body of the prosthesis is usually made of acrylic resin, which is radiolucent, but they include radiopaque metallic clips and hooks [16]. Thus, many prostheses can be determined on plain radiographs.

Various dislodged tubes (Fig. 6.6) may be detected in the gastrointestinal tract: A tube should be recognized to establish that it no longer serves its intended purpose, and because it may mimic other swallowed foreign objects.

Complications of dislodged or forgotten tubes include penetration, perforation (Fig. 6.7), and obstruction of the wall of the intestine (Fig. 6.8).

Stents used to overcome malignant biliary and gastrointestinal stenoses are made of plastic or metal. Stents to treat the latter, usually made of nitinol or stainless steel, can be bare, partially covered (at the center), or covered. The internal nonporous membrane prevents tumor growth through the mesh. Uncovered stents migrate less frequently, but they have significantly higher obstruction

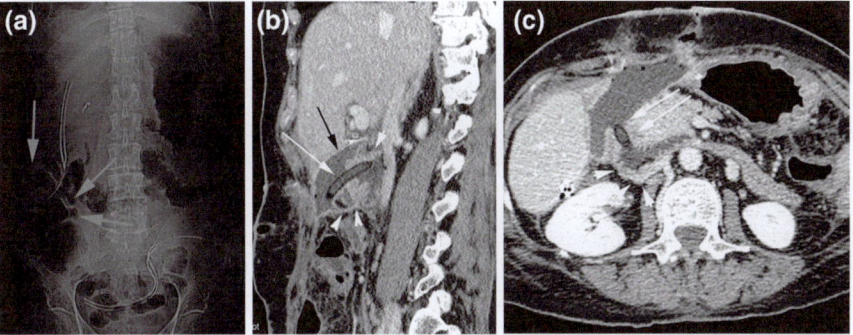

Fig. 6.6 Plain abdominal film **a** shows a transabdominal postoperation drainage tube (*white arrows*), located at the right lower abdominal quadrant. MDCT sagittal reformatted image **b** shows the drainage tube (*white arrow*) surrounded by a fluid collection (*black arrow*), passing through the duodenum inferior angle (*white arrowheads*). MDCT axial image **c** shows the drainage tube tip (*white arrows*) passing through the duodenum inferior angle (*white arrowheads*)

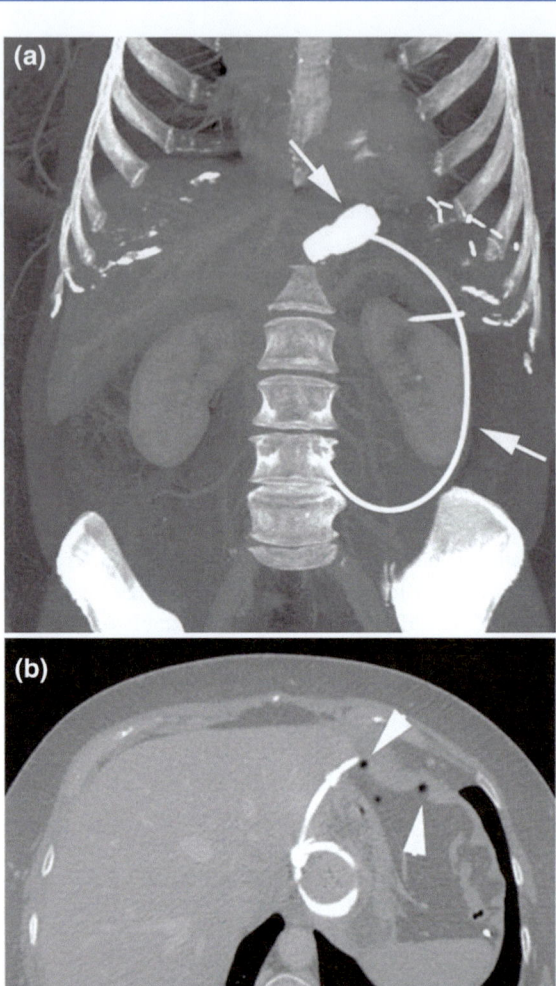

Fig. 6.7 MDCT, MIP coronal view **a** demonstrates a gastric bandage (*white arrow*). MDCT axial image **b** shows air bubbles entrapped in diaphragmatic tendons (*white arrowheads*), due to gastric bandage decubitus ulcer of the fundus

rates because of tumor ingrowth. Moreover, stents can be balloon expandable or, more frequently, self-expanding [17]. Stents may have a variable diameter and length. These devices can be placed during endoscopy through the viscus lumen or under fluoroscopic or endosonographic guidance through the viscus lumen or percutaneously [18, 19]. Stents may be deployed incorrectly or may dislodge after a variable interval of time after placement. Migration seems to occur more frequently with covered stents, probably because of their weaker anchorage, than

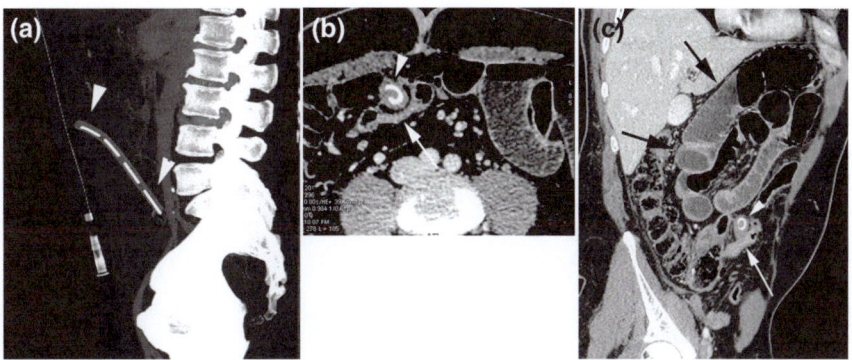

Fig. 6.8 MDCT, sagittal image **a** shows a surgical drainage tube forgotten in abdominal cavity (*white arrowheads*). MDCT axial image **b** demonstrates a fibrotic tissue around the tube (*white arrowhead*) joined to a closed small bowel loop (*white arrow*). MDCT oblique-coronal reformatted image **c** shows small bowel loops obstruction (*black arrows*), proximally to the closed small bowel loop (*white arrow*) and the tube (*white arrowhead*)

with uncovered stents. Stent migration may cause obstruction (Fig. 6.9), hemorrhage, and perforation (Fig. 6.10) [20, 21] or may have no consequence.

6.4 Considerations

Implanted devices are often seen in radiology practice. Radiologic evidence of correct locations of biliary and gastrointestinal stents is crucial for the treating physicians.

Biliary stents are commonly placed to treat biliary obstruction secondary to benign or malignant disease.

Fig. 6.9 MDCT, axial scan, shows a small bowel obstruction due to migration of an esophageal stent

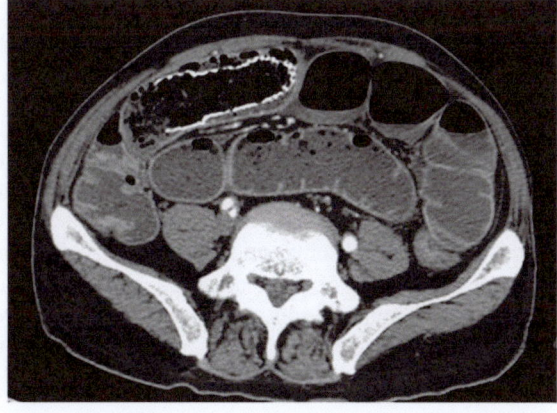

Fig. 6.10 Plain abdominal film **a** shows the presence of an endoprothesis (*white arrows*) inserted for the treatment of a gastric stenosis due to caustic fluid ingestion. MDCT axial image **b** demonstrates the gastric wall (*white arrowheads*), surrounded by multiple perigastric and perisplenic abscessed (*white arrows*) due to gastric prosthesis decubitus ulcer perforation

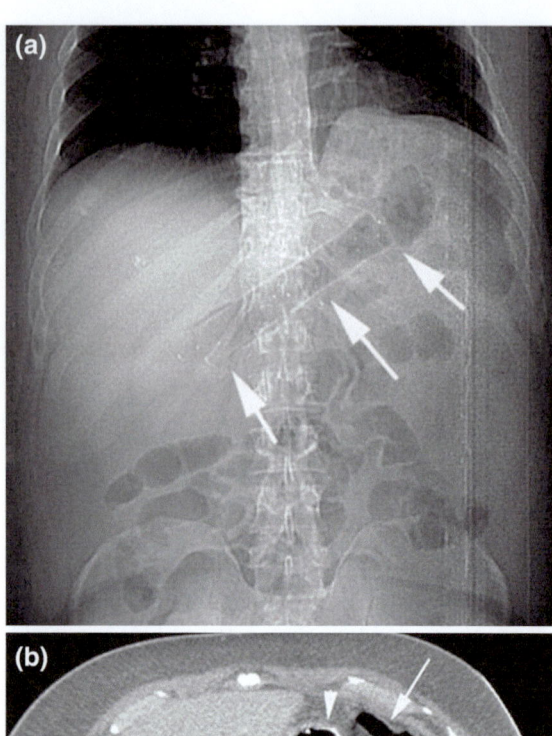

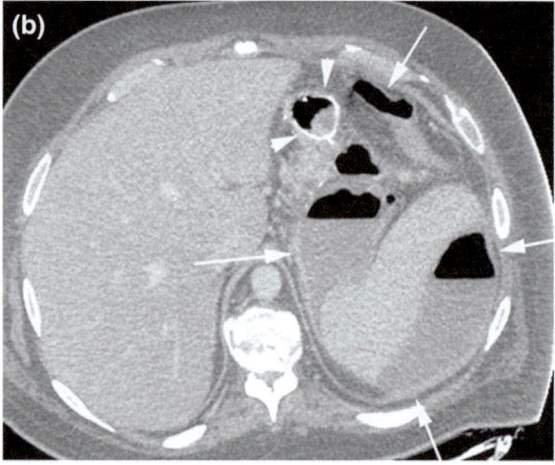

Malignant stenoses are more prone to most complications than benign stenoses, although the clinical failure of a stent procedure is not always caused by tumor-related factors [6]. Chemotherapy, antiangiogenic therapy, and radiation therapy may increase the likelihood that complications will develop [6].

In the literature, some studies emphasize the importance of recognizing the presence or absence of these devices—and of other devices such as endovascular catheters, pacemaker wires, genitourinary, and neurosurgical tubes—and how to evaluate their correct localization, understanding how they work, and identifying their complications [22].

Errors in interpretation of inserted devices such as catheters and enteric tubes are not very frequent. However, they have the potential to have a major impact on patient outcomes and management [23].

The checklist for radiologists interpreting images showing stents includes determining stent type, purpose, position, patency and integrity, and identifying persistent tissue (inflammation, free air, fluid or contrast material, enhancement, and bleeding) if present [23].

MDCT has distinct advantages in comparison with endoscopic procedures and conventional radiographic studies for visualizing the presence of stents and diagnosing potential associated complications. MDCT provides high-resolution images related not only to the stent, but also to the wall of the biliary or enteric segment where the stent is located and supplies crucial information related to the surrounding fat planes, organs, and structures. In fact, whereas endoscopy and conventional radiologic studies show only intraluminal changes, MDCT depicts extraluminal signs of complications (such as free peritoneal air, retroperitoneal gas, or fluid collections) [24].

6.5 Conclusions

Despite various systems and safeguards available, unintentionally retained surgically placed foreign bodies remain difficult to eliminate completely. Developing a standardized approach to the request, "intraoperative film, rule out foreign body," is essential to reduce the adverse outcomes associated with this problem.

Patients with gastrointestinal symptoms with known stents should be thoroughly worked up for the pathology requiring stent placement, as well as for the possibility of stent migration. The incorrect position of a misplaced or displaced stent is frequently overlooked, especially when the patient is asymptomatic. However, prompt recognition of misplaced or displaced stents is important because percutaneous or endoscopic repositioning or removal of the device can be performed before irreversible injuries develop.

MDCT allows an accurate diagnosis in terms of the location (i.e., intraluminal or extraluminal) and nature of a misplaced or displaced stent. Inspection of the scout image may often be helpful and should be an integral part of the imaging evaluation. Biliary and gastrointestinal stents must be differentiated from other foreign bodies that may be found within the lumen of the gastrointestinal tract.

References

1. Chun HJ, Kim ES, Hyun JJ et al (2010) Gastrointestinal and biliary stents. J Gastroenterol Hepatol 25:234–243
2. Katsanos K, Sabharwal T, Adam A (2010) Stenting of the upper gastrointestinal tract: current status. Cardiovasc Intervent Radiol 33:690–705

3. Baerlocher MO, Asch MR, Vellahottam A et al (2008) Safety and efficacy of gastrointestinal stents in cancer patients at a community hospital. Can J Surg 51:130–134
4. Kim JH, Song H-Y, Shin JH et al (2007) Stent collapse as a delayed complication of placement of a covered gastroduodenal stent. AJR 188:1495–1499
5. Kullman E, Frozanpor F, Söderlund C et al (2010) Covered versus uncovered self-expandable nitinol stents in the palliative treatment of malignant distal biliary obstruction: results from a randomized, multicenter study. Gastrointest Endosc 72:915–923
6. Fernández-Esparrach G, Bordas JM, Giráldez MD et al (2010) Severe complications limit long-term clinical success of self-expanding metal stents in patients with obstructive colorectal cancer. Am J Gastroenterol 105:1087–1093
7. Diller R, Senninger N, Kautz G et al (2003) Stent migration necessitating surgical intervention. Surg Endosc 17:1803–1807
8. Namdar T, Raffel AM, Topp SA et al (2007) Complications and treatment of migrated biliary endoprostheses: a review of the literature. World J Gastroenterol 13:5397–5399
9. Johanson J, Schmalg M, Greenor J (1992) Incidence and risk factors for biliary and pancreatic stent migration. Gastrointest Endosc 38:341–346
10. Jendresen MB, Svendsen LB (2001) Proximal displacement of biliary stent with distal perforation and impaction in the pancreas. Endoscopy 33:195
11. Liebich-Bartholain L, Kleinau U, Elsbernd H et al (2001) Biliary pneumonitis after proximal stent migration. Gastrointest Endosc 2001:382–384
12. Pathak AK, de Souza LJ (2001) Duodenocolic fistula: an unusual sequela of stent migration. Endoscopy 33:731
13. Ruffolo TA, Lehman GA, Sherman S et al (1992) Biliary stent migration with colonic diverticular impaction. Gastrointest Endosc 38:81–83
14. Gayer G, Petrovitch I, Jeffrey RB (2011) Foreign objects encountered in the abdominal cavity at CT. Radiographics 31:409–428
15. Abdullah BJ, Teong LK, Mahadevan J et al (1998) Dental prosthesis ingested and impacted in the esophagus and orolaryngopharynx. J Otolaryngol 27:190–194
16. Nwafo DC, Anyanwu CH, Egbue MO (1980) Impacted esophageal foreign bodies of dental origin. Ann Otol Rhinol Laryngol 89:129–131
17. Gwon DI, Ko GY, Kim JH et al (2010) A comparative analysis of PTFE-covered and uncovered stents for palliative treatment of malignant extrahepatic biliary obstruction. AJR 195:W463–W469
18. Kang SG (2010) Gastrointestinal stent update. Gut Liver 4(suppl 1):S19–S24
19. Horaguchi J, Fujita N, Noda Y et al (2009) Endosonography-guided biliary drainage in cases with difficult transpapillary endoscopic biliary drainage. Dig Endosc 21:239–244
20. Görich J, Rilinger N, Krämer S et al (1997) Displaced metallic biliary stents: technique and rationale for interventional radiologic retrieval. AJR 169:1529–1533
21. Kim HC, Han JK, Kim TK et al (2000) Duodenal perforation as a delayed complication of placement of an esophageal stent. J Vasc Interv Radiol 11:902–904
22. Hunter TB, Taljanovic MS, Tsau PH et al (2004) Medical devices of the chest. Radiographics 24:1725–1746
23. Fuentealba I, Taylor GA (2012) Diagnostic errors with inserted tubes, lines and catheters in children. Pediatr Radiol 42:1305–1315
24. Catalano O, De Bellis M, Sandomenico F et al (2012) Complications of biliary and gastrointestinal stents: MDCT of the cancer patient. AJR 199:W187–W196

Intravascular Foreign Bodies

7

Raffaella Niola, Sergio Capece, Mario Fusari
and Franco Maglione

7.1 Introduction

In recent years, interest in endovascular foreign bodies (IFB) has greatly increased, as evidenced by the increasingly high casuistry and the growing number of publications on this subject. Surely the increase in interventional procedures can be correlated either as the cause, due to the increasingly higher number of IFB iatrogenic, or to the increasing introduction into clinical practice of a number of techniques for the recovery of these.

Although much has been written on the recovery of IFB, as regards imaging in the literature there are no clear guidelines. A first classification can be based on strictly radiological differentiation between foreign bodies that are radio-opaque and non radio-opaque. However, the small number of reported cases of non radio-opaque foreign bodies makes us lean toward a disquisition based on two main aspects, namely iatrogenic and noniatrogenic.

7.2 Iatrogenic Intravascular Foreign Bodies

In the last 20 years, the number of minimally invasive and interventional techniques involving the implantation and use of intravascular objects has rapidly increased, and the incidence of a lost intravascular foreign body (IFB) is becoming a more frequent clinical problem [1, 2]. A large number of iatrogenic IFBs most commonly described in the literature are embolized central line fragments, followed by guide wires, catheter fragments, embolization coils, inferior vena cava

---

R. Niola (✉) · S. Capece · M. Fusari · F. Maglione
Vascular and Interventional Radiology, Cardarelli Hospital, Naples, Italy
e-mail: raffaellaniola@tiscali.it

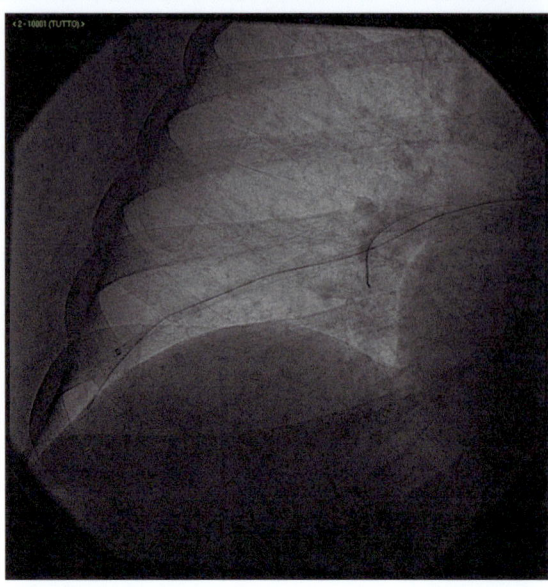

Fig. 7.1 Guide wire displaced in right pulmonary artery

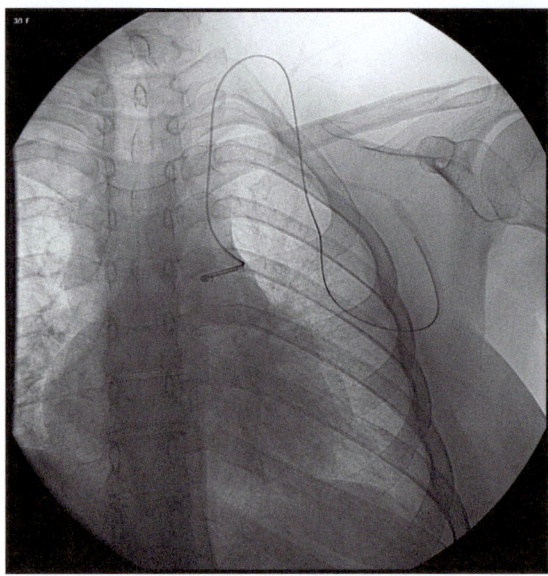

Fig. 7.2 Central venous catheter displaced in left subclavian vein

filters, cardiac valve fragments, sheaths, pacing wires, and occluder devices [1] Figs. 7.1 and 7.2.

The major causes of intravascular catheter embolization were catheter injury during explantation, pinch-off syndrome, catheter disconnection, and catheter rupture [3–5]. Poor guide catheter/guide wire support, proximal vessel tortuosity,

Fig. 7.3 Broken pacemaker electrodus in left subclavian vein

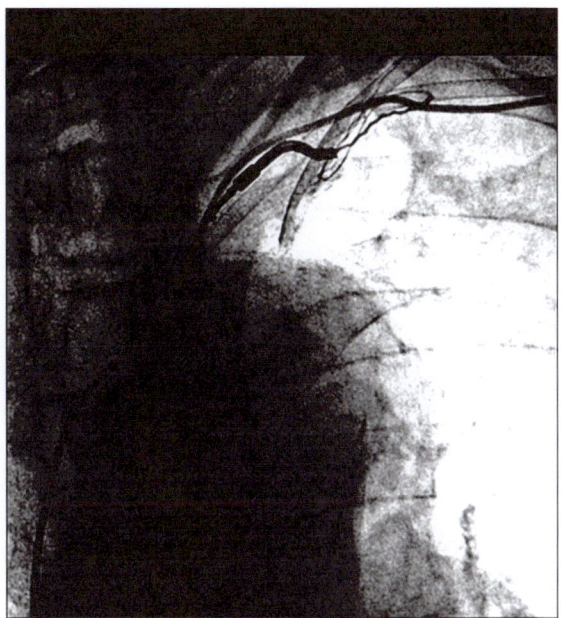

and vessel calcification are risk factors that can result in device (e.g., stent) loss (Figs. 7.3 and 7.4).

In addition to faults and manufacturing defects, a high proportion of lost IFBs result from technical error and the lack of experience on the part of the operator. As we can find in the literature, the majority of migrated lines have resulted from tunneled catheters being inappropriately cut by inexperienced staff at the time of attempted line removal. To avoid this complication, good training and knowledge of the devices being used is essential. Good case planning with appropriate equipment in the range of the operator's experience and training will be helpful.

Particular mention is required of portacath implanted in the subclavian vein, a location that carries a particular catheter injury risk, exposing them to greater total repetitive traumatic injury and risk of fragmentation. The most common location of the catheter fracture is the infraclavicular region secondary to the so-called pinch-off syndrome or thoracic inlet syndrome. Previous data suggest that material fatigue may play a key role in catheter fracture [6].

The first step in IFB research is an accurate medical history of the patient; it is necessary to have information about the type of catheter, the shape, size, and the possible location of the object.

Depending on the type of catheter and its primitive location, the first diagnostic orientation should be based on its possible presence in the arterial, venous, or pulmonary vessels. In fact, on the basis that most IFBs are fragments of devices, their detachment follows an embolization in the direction of blood flow, in almost all cases. For these reasons, for central venous catheters and peripheral venous

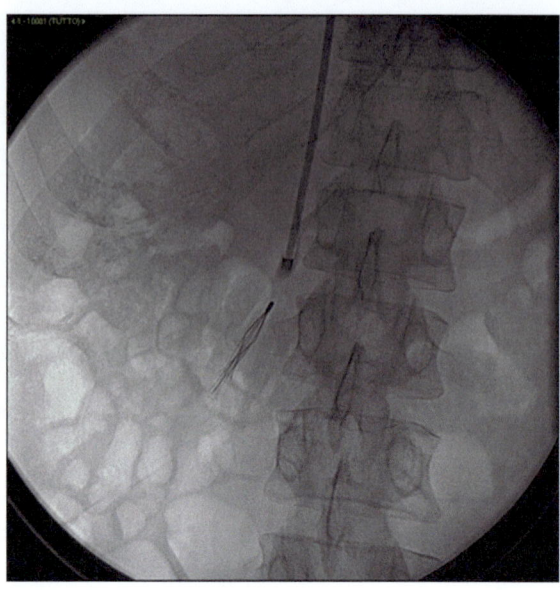

Fig. 7.4 Vena cava filter opened in the hepatic vein

catheters the vessels of probable location will be the central veins, the right heart, and the pulmonary circulation, while for IFBs that originate in an artery we have to turn our attention to a possible peripheral embolization.

As regards imaging, plain film is the first-line investigation followed by fluoroscopy. Catheter fragments are generally fluoroscopically poorly visible because they are small and are made of material that poorly attenuates X-rays. Overlying tissues and movement-related artifacts (e.g., cardiac motion) further reduce fluoroscopic image clarity. Some authors suggest to use computed tomography (CT) as a first-line investigation, but we have to consider the higher risk of radiation exposure for the patient []. Catheter fragments may be very small, and it could be hard to identify them even on CT. Magnetic resonance imaging (MRI) is done when we are sure that the foreign body is known to be MRI compatible in cases of peripheral embolization. In the case of metallic lost IFBs, a gradient echo sequence will result in susceptibility artifacts. Ultrasound, sometimes, can be helpful in detachment. To avoid further device migration, once localized, the interval to subsequent attempted device retrieval should be minimized.

7.3 Noniatrogenic Intravascular Foreign Bodies

The majority of noniatrogenic intravascular foreign bodies consist in gunshot bullets.

A bullet embolus should be suspected in any patient who has a gunshot wound without an exit wound, when the signs and symptoms do not correlate with those expected from the suspected course of the missile, and when radiological investigations show that missile location deviates from the path of penetration [7, 8]. Bullet emboli access the vascular system by direct propulsion or erosion into the vessel lumen. Eighty percent are arterial in nature with only 20 % being venous. Arterial embolization is symptomatic (claudication, peripheral ischemia, and thrombophlebitis) in 80 % of cases, and typically originates from the pulmonary artery, heart, or great vessels with embolization to peripheral vessels causing limb ischemia, particularly in the lower extremities. Venous embolization is symptomatic (dyspnea, haemoptysis, and chest pain) in 30 % of cases, with embolization from the large peripheral veins, vena cava or liver, to the right side of the heart, particularly the right ventricle or pulmonary arteries [8].

There are two rare documented subgroups of embolization. First is retrograde embolization seen in 15 % of venous cases and defined as projectile movement against the normal direction of blood flow. Second is paradoxical embolization, defined as the passage of a foreign body from the venous to the arterial system by communication through a right to left shunt. Causes include arteriovenous fistula, atrioventricular perforation, ventricular septal defect, or patent foramen ovale [9]. Diagnosis of foreign body emboli is through X-ray, computerized tomography, and echocardiography.

Unlike iatrogenic embolization, the traumatic patient hemodynamically stable undergoes an evaluation of imaging by CT in almost all cases. So CT is often the first method used. However, repeated X-ray examination is the best method for an accurate assessment of possible vascular migration of missile. Even in these cases ultrasound can demonstrate the hyperechoic IFB with the characteristic trailing band of increased echogenicity (comet tail) [10].

The MRI is strictly contraindicated for the magnetic nature of bullet.

7.4 IFB Retrieval

The first case of IFB was documented in 1954 [11], the case report detailing a CVC found in the right atrium of a patient during autopsy. A few years later, in 1964 [12], Thomas described the first percutaneous retrieval, through a bronchoscopic forceps, of an IFB, a fragment of guide wire migrated into the right atrium. The technique was quickly adopted as an alternative to surgical removal and nowadays the percutaneous intravascular recovery is considered the "gold standard" [13]. Key factors to achieve a successful outcome are appropriate knowledge of the equipment available, the different techniques, and obviously the operator experience. We have already considered the need for careful imaging to detect the foreign body and also planning the procedure to minimize the risks connected. The presence of the anesthesiologist is important, as in any interventional procedure, to ensure the right management of the patient [13]. It is also necessary to adequately inform the patient about the procedure, the risks associated, and the possible alternative treatments [14]. It is essential to have in one's arsenal, ready for use, all necessary devices such as snares, intravascular forceps, sheaths of various sizes, guide wires, various shaped catheters, and occlusion balloons. Previous planning can optimize the procedure choosing the best way to go.

7.5 Removal Techniques and Devices

The loop snare is frequently the first choice device for the removal of an IFB. The modern design allows the loop to emerge at 90° to the catheter facilitating by far the tracking of the loop and then the capture of IFB. There are snare loops of various sizes, including microsnares (e.g., Radius Medical) from 2 gauges up to 35 mm (Gooseneck, EV3, Welter retrieval loop, Cook, Trefoil ensnare/TriSnare Merit Medical). All models of loop snares are designed on the same principle: the use of moveable nitinol wire loop which passes through a guiding catheter. The snares have an excellent safety profile, are relatively atraumatic, simple to use, and effective even in less experienced hands [13, 15].

7.6 Proximal Capture Technique

This is the basic technique when using a loop snare. It is necessary to use a loop snare of a size appropriate to the vessel; i.e., the fully open loop must be of a size equal to or slightly smaller than the vessel where the IFB is located [13, 16]. The snare loop proceeds to the target vessel on a previously positioned guide wire. When the snare is in position within the target vessel the external catheter is withdrawn allowing the loop to fully open within the vessel lumen. The whole system is then advanced to positioning the open loop around the IFB, or around a specific part of it. Now the loop is closed by advancing the catheter to tighten the IFB. When the complete control of IFB occurs, the entire system, along with the IFB, is pulled back into the sheath. To be successful, a free end on the IFB is needed. On the contrary, there are two options: either the approach from a different direction, or the use of a shaped catheter like an SOS Omni or a balloon that can be used to stop, move, or bend the IFB to allow the access to a free end of the same. When the snare holds the IFB, this one could lie perpendicularly: if it is a floppy one, no problem occurs because it folds into half [13]; however, in case of a stiff one, a risk of damage or vessel perforation could happen. Thus, it is better to grasp the IFB at one end; its natural motion will help to keep the body aligned with the axis of the vessel [17]. Even when the vessel is prepared, recovery may be difficult. To facilitate the recovery a second snare can be used from another intravascular access to apply a rotational force on IFB [13, 16, 18] (Fig. 7.5).

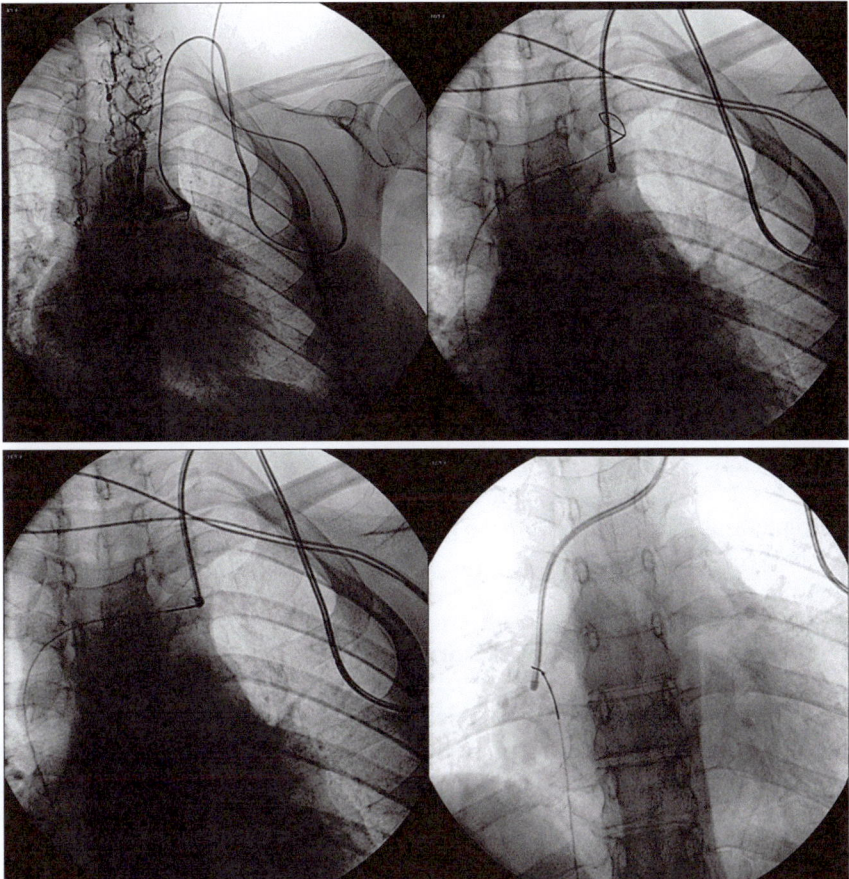

Fig. 7.5 Retrieval of CVC in subclavian vein by loop snare (Gooseneck, EV3) with proximal capture technique

7.7 Distal Capture Technique

The approach to distal capture may be attempted if a guide wire can pass through the IFB (e.g., a guide wire as the Super Stiff Amplatz). A micro snare is used to create a road along the side of IFB and beyond it; then the micro snare loop is used to capture the end of the guide wire that crosses the IFB. In this way the IFB is captured between the guide wire and the snare catheter and remains absolutely aligned with the vessel.

7.8 Coaxial Snare Technique

This technique uses a guide wire and a snare to reduce the angle between a foreign body, the snare, and the sheath, and can be used with tubular foreign bodies. The purpose is to pass the guide wire through the lumen of the IFB; the snare is placed around the guide wire which looks like a rail to guide the loop snare distally. At the proximal pole of the tubular IFB the loop snare opens and captures the IFB along the guide wire. This is now trapped within the loop snare and a traction can be used to torque and drive the proximal pole of the IFB into the sheath [19].

7.9 Lateral Capture Technique

This is a variation of the distal capture technique, by which approach the snare opens distally to IFB. A rigid guide wire is passed around the IFB but from the opposite side of snare and then through the loop of the snare; so, the loop is closed and captures the guide wire. Both the guide wire and the catheter snare tighten the IFB between their arms.

Stone Retrieval Baskets and Dormia Baskets

The Dormiabasket is a well-known device often used in the biliary system. Two nitinol loops wire spirales can be spread when releasing without significant risk of damage to the vessel wall. The device provides goodhaptic feedback and small caliber (-3 F) that can go into a thin guide catheter and have access to small vessels [13, 16, 20].The disadvantage of baskets is poor navigation; Dormia also have a very stiff end that could create a risk of damage to the endothelium.

7.10 Balloon Catheter Technique

The technique of the balloon is useful in the recovery of stents; it requires a guide wire passing through the IFB or a portion of it. The same guide wire can then be used to guide a low-profile balloon catheter inside or distally to the lost IFB. It is important to choose an appropriate retrieval balloon: if too large, it will not pass the IFB and could push it distally; if too small, when inflated, it will not capture the IFB. The balloon must be inflated into the stent at low pressure, to engage the stent without expanding it. If the balloon is deployed distally to the IFB, it must be gently pulled back up to engage the IFB; the entire unit can be now withdrawn into the sheath or into a fit proximal retrieval area. If the IFB cannot be retrieved in a sheath, the balloon can be inflated to block the IFB in an easily approachable surgical site. The technique of the small balloon may be used in addition to the loop snare to facilitate the gripping of the loop on the stent. The loop snare is positioned around the proximal part of the PTA balloon which is then inflated near the stent. This leads the snare loop in alignment with the stent. The snare can be advanced over the balloon and the stent, and used to capture both the balloon and the stent, or to slide the stent over the guide wire [21].

7.11 Guide Wire as a Snare

A guide wire can be used with a catheter to build a loop snare homemade shaping the tip of the guide wire in pig-tail so that it twirls IFB.

7.12 Hairpin Capture Technique

Technique that involves the bending of a thin guide wire (e.g. guide wire 0.010 or 0014 inch) to form a hairpin and is then inserted into a guide catheter and passed through the stent, so that when pulled back it captures the IFB at its distal end [22].

7.13 Two-Wire Technique

By the two-wire technique a guide wire is passed through the lumen of the stent and another stiffer guide wire is passed through the struts of the stent. The guides are held together with a twisting motion and rotation along their axis as long as the rotation of the twisted wires reaches the lost stent. This wire strand produces enough force to capture the stent and allows retrieval from the vessel [22] (Fig. 7.6).

7.14 Intravascular Retrieval Forceps and Biliary or Myocardial Biopsy Forceps

Intravascular dedicated forceps are now available in a large variety of designs. They have side opening jaws, pass inside guide catheters, and have guide wires to assist the maneuver; the range of sizes varies from 12 to 3 F. The advantage of the forceps is they do not need a free end for the retrieval of IFB. These devices have a quite high iatrogenic risk and must be used judiciously [23–25] (Fig. 7.7).

7.15 Miscellanea

Incorrect opening of a vena cava filter in the hepatic vein occurs rarely. In this case a dedicated "cone of recovery" of the same filter can be used to remove it from the incorrect side (Fig. 7.7).

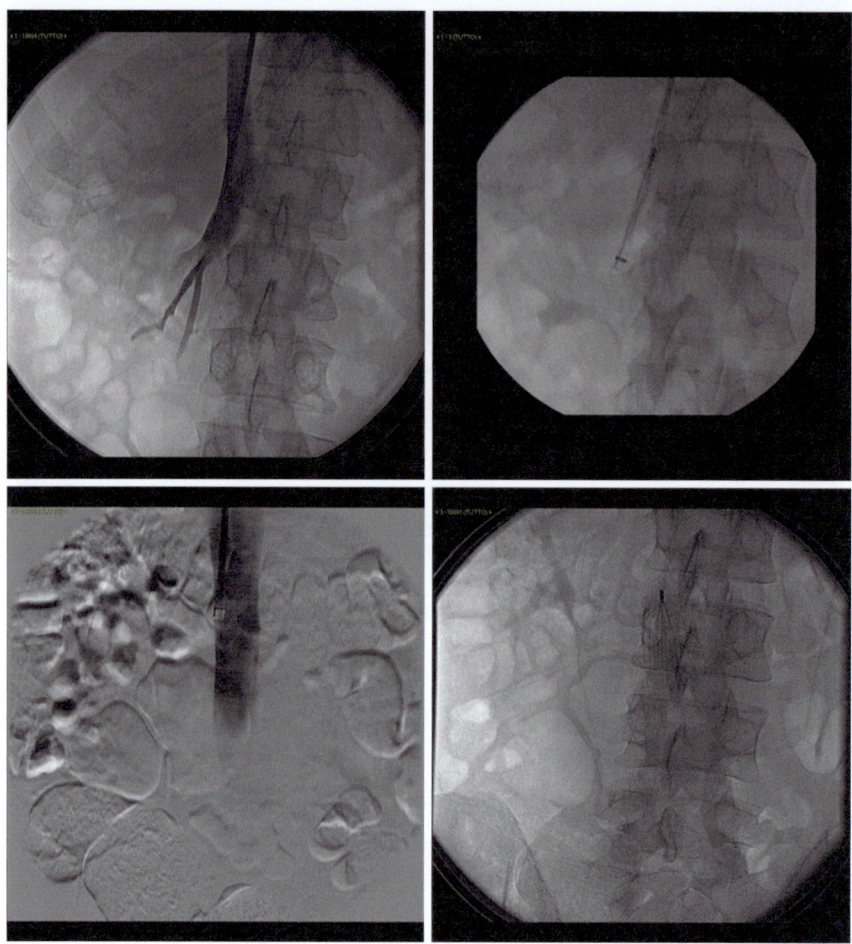

Fig. 7.6 Retrieval of vena cava filter accidentally opened in the hepatic vein

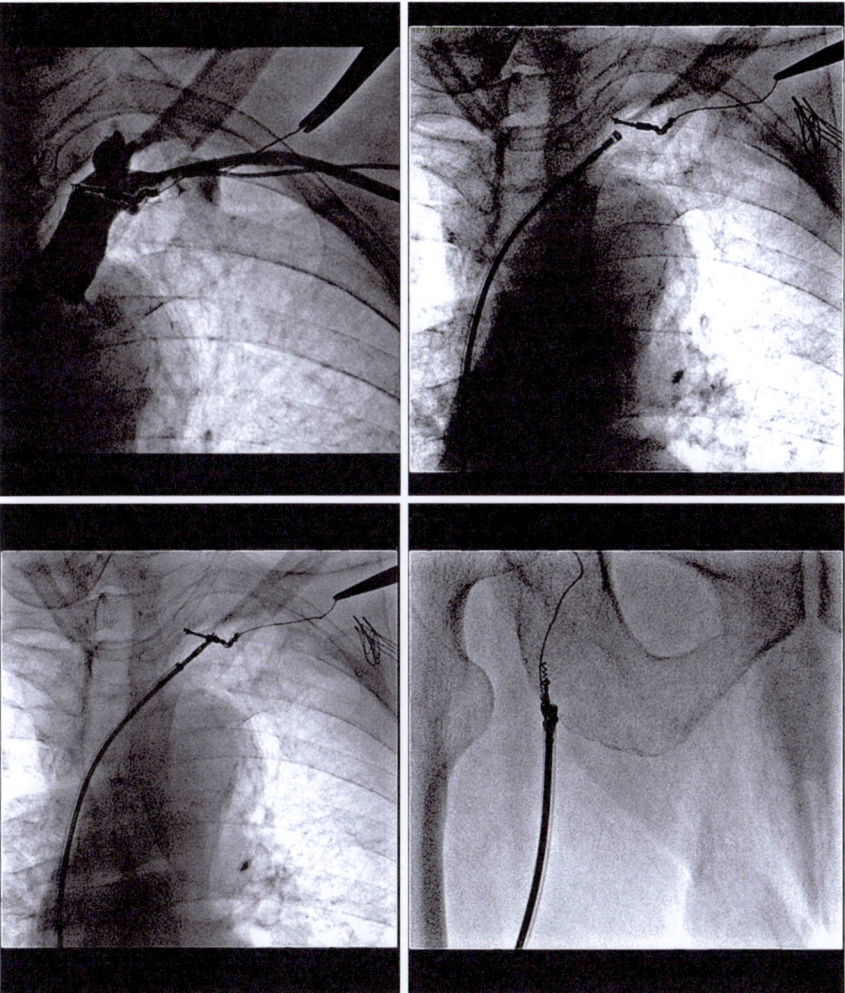

Fig. 7.7 Retrieval of pacemaker electrode in subclavian vein by alligator forceps and stopped in femoral vein. The IFB was then surgically removed

References

1. Wolf F, Schernthaner RE, Dirisamer A et al (2008) Endovascular management of lost or misplaced intravascular objects: experiences of 12 years. Cardiovasc Intervent Radiol 31(3):563–568. PubMed PMID: 17955287
2. Woodhouse JB, Uberoi R (2012) Techniques for intravascular foreign body retrieval. Cardiovasc Intervent Radiol. PubMed PMID: 23073559
3. Egglin TK, Dickey KW, Rosenblatt M, Pollak JS (1995) Retrieval of intravascular foreign bodies: experience in 32 cases. AJR Am J Roentgenol 164(5):1259–1264

4. Morse SS, Strauss EB, Hashim SW et al (1986) Percutaneous retrieval of an unusually large, nonopaque intravascular foreign body. AJR Am J Roentgenol 146(4):863–864. PubMed PMID: 3485361
5. Surov A, Wienke A, Carter JM et al (2009) Intravascular embolization of venous catheter–causes, clinical signs, and management: a systematic review. JPEN J Parenter Enteral Nutr 33(6):677–685. PubMed PMID: 19675301
6. Çilingiroğlu M, Akkuş Nl (2012) Embolization of a PORT-A-CATH device in the main pulmonary artery and its percutaneous extraction in a patient with pinch-off syndrome. Turk Kardiyol Dern Ars 40(2):162–164. doi: 10.5543/tkda.2012.01821. PubMed PMID: 22710588
7. Demirkilic U, Yilmaz AT, Tatar H, Ozturk OY (2004) Bullet embolism to the pulmonary artery. Interact Cardiovasc Thorac Surg. 3(2):356–358
8. Greaves N (2010) Gunshot bullet embolus with pellet migration from the leftbrachiocephalic vein to the right ventricle: a case report. Scand J Trauma Resusc Emerg Med 18:36. doi: 10.1186/1757-7241-18-36. PubMed PMID:20565913; PubMed Central PMCID: PMC2898681
9. Bining HJ, Artho GP, Vuong PD, Evans DC, Powell T (2007) Venous bullet embolism to the right ventricle. Br J Radiol 80(960):e296–e298
10. Bonk RT, Harrison SD, Meissner MH (1996) Intravascular bullet localization by sonography. AJR Am J Roentgenol 167(1):152
11. Turner DD, Sommers SC (1954) Accidental passage of a polyethylene catheter from cubital vein to right atrium; report of a fatal case. N Engl J Med 251:744–745
12. Thomas J, Sinclair-Smith B, Bloomfield D, Davachi A (1964) Non-surgical retrieval of a broken segment of steel spring guide from the right atrium and inferior vena cava. Circulation 30:106–108
13. Techniques for Intravascular Foreign Body Retrieval Joe B. Woodhouse Raman Uberoi. Cardiovasc Intervent Radiol. doi: 10.1007/s00270-012-0488-8
14. Alexandre M, Sebastin T, Vikramaditya P (2009) Combinedsurgical and endovascular retrieval of a migrated rigid mitral valve ring. J Vasc Interv Radiol 20:1101–1102
15. Mallmann CV, Wolf KJ, Wacker FK (2008) Retrieval of vascular foreign bodies using a self-made wire snare. Acta Radiol 49:1124–1128
16. Wolf F, Schernthaner RE, Dirisamer A et al (2008) Endovascular management of lost or misplaced intravascular objects: experiences of 12 years. Cardiovasc Intervent Radiol 31:563
17. Guimaraes M, Denton CE, Uflacker R et al (2012) Percutaneous retrieval of an Amplatzer septal occluder device that had migrated to the aortic arch. Cardiovasc Intervent Radiol 35:430–433
18. Seong CK, Kim YJ, Chung JW et al (2002) Tubular foreign body or stent: safe retrieval or repositioning using the coaxial snare technique. Korean J Radiol 3:30–37
19. Sheth R, Someshwar V, Warawdekar G (2007) Percutaneous retrieval of misplaced intravascular foreign objects with the Dormia basket: an effective solution. Cardiovasc Intervent Radiol 30:48–53
20. Cishek MB, Laslett L, Gershony G (1995) Balloon catheter retrieval of dislodged coronary artery stents: a novel technique. Cathet Cardiovasc Diagn 34:350–352
21. Eeckhout E, Stauffer JC, Goy JJ (1993) Retrieval of a migrated coronary stent by means of an alligator forceps catheter. Cathet Cardiovasc Diagn 30:166–168
22. Brilakis ES, Best PJ, Elesber AA et al (2005) Incidence, retrieval methods, and outcomes of stent loss during percutaneous coronary intervention: a large single-center experience. Catheter Cardiovasc Interv 66:333–340
23. Yeung LY, Hastings GS, Alexander JQ (2010) Endovascular retrieval of inferior vena cava filter penetrating into aorta: an unusual presentation of abdominal pain. Vasc Endovascular Surg 44:683–686
24. Schroeder ME, Pryor HI 2nd, Chun AK et al (2011) Retrograde migration and endovascular retrieval of a venous bullet embolus. J Vasc Surg 53:1113–1115

25. Berder V, Bedossa M, Gras D et al (1993) Retrieval of a lost coronary stent from the descending aorta using a PTCA balloon and biopsy forceps. Cathet Cardiovasc Diagn 28:351–353
26. Boersma D, van Strijen MJ, Kloppenburg GT et al (2012) Endovascular retrieval of a dislodged femoral arterial closure device with alligator forceps. J Vasc Surg 55:1150–1152
27. Struck MF, Kaden I, Heiser A, Steen M (2008) Cross-over endovascular retrieval of a lost guide wire from the subclavian vein. J Vasc Access 9:304–306

Foreign Bodies as Complications of Endovascular Devices

Antonio Pinto, Stefania Daniele and Luigia Romano

8.1 Introduction

A wide number of intravascular devices exists, and new devices are constantly being introduced. Nevertheless, the preponderance of devices observed in everyday practice have been used for a number of years, and many of the newest devices are variations on a topic.

Central venous catheters (CVCs) are used to supply temporary or long-term vascular access. They are valuable in the management of various conditions, such as those requiring regular blood sampling, total parenteral nutrition, chemotherapy, and long-term antibiotics. There are many complications associated with the insertion and maintenance of CVCs: one of them is the presence of intravascular foreign body.

Angioplasty and stenting of femoral, iliac, renal, and coronary arterial lesions are common: well-known complications of these stents include intimal dissection, thrombosis, malpositioning, infections, and rupture. Foreign bodies as complication of vascular devices may also involve patients submitted to endovascular repair of abdominal aortic aneurysm.

A. Pinto (✉) · S. Daniele · L. Romano
Department of Diagnostic Radiological Imaging, Cardarelli Hospital,
Via A. Cardarelli 9, 80131, Naples, Italy
e-mail: antopin1968@libero.it

S. Daniele
e-mail: cheops@tin.it

L. Romano
e-mail: luigia.romano@fastwebnet.it

8.2 Central Venous Catheters

A large spectrum of central venous access procedures are performed in the world every year. This number is increasing as the indications and applications are expanded. These include hemodynamic monitoring, fluid replacement, hemodialysis, total parenteral nutrition, delivery of blood products and drugs such as vasopressors, chemotherapy, and antibiotics. CVCs may be classified into four groups: (1) peripherally inserted central catheters (PICCs), (2) temporary (nontunnelled) CVCs, (3) permanent (tunnelled) CVCs, and (4) implantable ports. The type of catheter chosen is primarily based on its proposed function and duration of use [1].

Central venous catheters are among the most ubiquitous of medical devices used in hospitalized patients from the very sick to those who are minimally ill. They should be radiopaque for easy visibility on routine radiographs. Unfortunately, there are still some poorly opacified catheters that are difficult to identify without an adequate quality chest radiograph and without a proper history of catheter insertion or use.

CVCs inserted into the subclavian vein or into the internal jugular vein have been the standard approach for central line placement for the past 30 years.

Although CVCs have been in clinical use for many years, there is still significant debate as to what represents optimal practice in terms of method of placement and minimization of procedure-related complications.

Placing CVCs entails risk. The rate of major and minor complications can be as high as 10 %. This depends on operator experience, access site, patient's clinical conditions, presence of vascular anatomic variants, coagulation status, and previous catheterizations [1]. Complications include pneumothorax, malpositioning, great vessel and cardiac perforation, inadvertent arterial puncture, fibrin sheath formation, catheter-related central venous thrombosis, and intravascular foreign bodies.

Pneumothorax is amongst the most prevalent immediate complications of unguided CVCs insertion. It occurs more commonly with subclavian puncture than with internal jugular vein puncture [2].

The published incidence of pneumothorax ranges from 0–3.3 % with radiological placement of tunneled CVCs [3, 4]. Pneumothorax is a potentially life-threatening complication, which may require placement of a chest drain. Luckily, most pneumothoraces associated with CVCs remain asymptomatic. Usually, this complication is evident on a post-procedural chest radiograph, but may occasionally manifest several days after CVCs placement [5].

Although uncommon, malpositioning of the CVCs may occur, and are associated with serious sequelae. Knowledge of normal and variant venous anatomy is crucial for catheter positioning. If fluoroscopy is not used during catheter insertion, a malpositioned catheter may lie in the internal jugular vein, contra-lateral subclavian or axillary vein, internal mammary vein, or left superior accessory vein.

Catheter perforation of the great vessels and heart is uncommon with an overall incidence less than 1 % [6] but is associated with significant morbidity and mortality. The catheter tip position within the pericardial reflection is associated with increased risk of cardiac perforation and tamponade [7].

Inadvertent arterial punctures during CVCs insertion occurs in up to 3 % [8]. Significant morbidity and death has also been reported. Catheters deployed using conventional landmarks may lacerate the subclavian, carotid or external iliac arteries, or rarely be incorrectly inserted into these arteries.

Another complication of CVCs insertion is fibrin sheath formation which is the most common cause of catheter dysfunction. Fibrin sheath formation usually occurs in patients with long-term catheters, such as those undergoing hemodialysis, and refers to a proteinaceous coat composed of eosinophilic material and inflammatory cells that envelop the catheter from insertion site to tip [9].

Central venous thrombosis is a well-recognized complication of CVC (Fig. 8.1), with an overall incidence between 30 and 70 % [10, 11]. Thrombosis occurs where there has been repeated trauma to the endothelium from the catheter tip [12]. There is a relationship between high placement of the catheter tip (upper SVC or above) and thrombosis [12, 13].

Catheter-related thrombosis can be intraluminal or periluminal. Several factors influence the formation of catheter-related venous thrombosis including catheter duration, the caliber of the catheter, the access vein used, or systemic comorbidities [14]. Although most thrombosis is either asymptomatic or results in catheter blockage alone, serious life-threatening vascular events, including SVC syndrome and pulmonary embolism may occur.

The common sources of intravascular foreign body (Fig. 8.2) are lost guidewires during insertion and catheter fractures related to tearing of the catheter during insertion or following catheter damage during removal or traction on the catheter-hub junction. Fracture of CVCs is a rare but serious complication of their use.

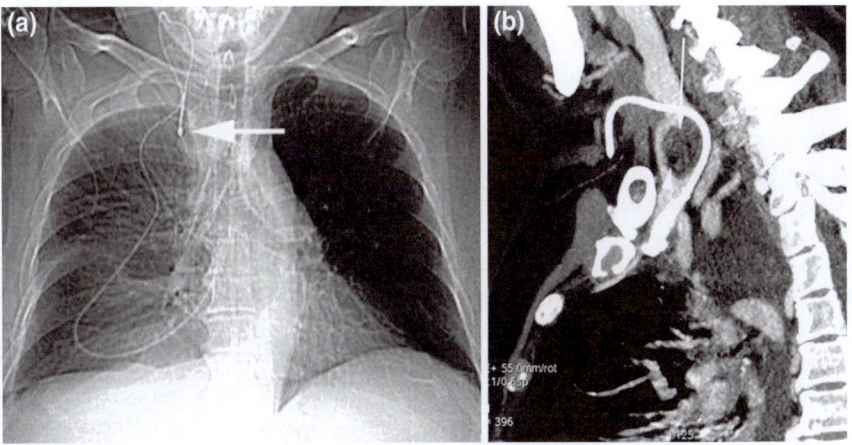

Fig. 8.1 Plain chest film **a** shows a central venous catheter positioned in the superior vena cava (*arrow*). MDCT sagittal reformatted image **b** shows a large infectious thrombus (*arrow*) mixed to air bubble (*arrowhead*) in the superior vena cava lumen, closed to the catheter

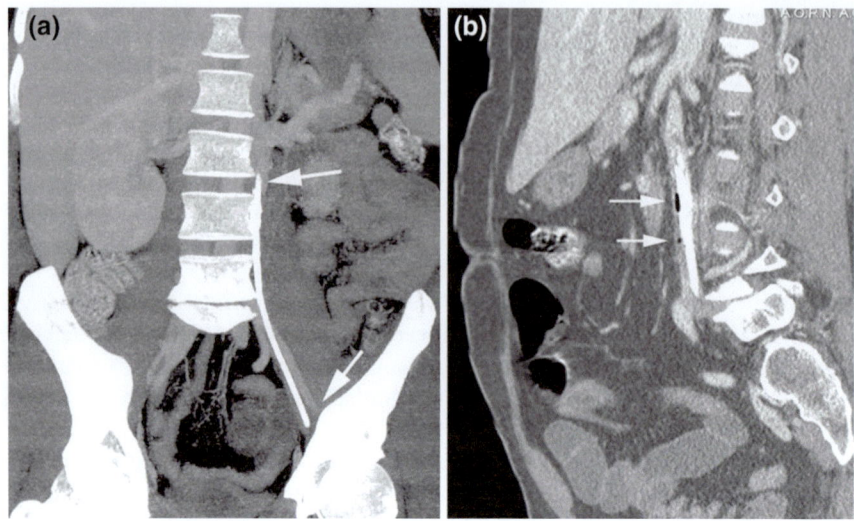

Fig. 8.2 MDCT coronal reformatted image **a** shows a long venous catheter fragment at the *left* paravertebral side. MDCT sagittal reformatted image **b** reveals the presence of a large infectious venous catheter fragment surrounded by air bubbles (*arrows*) in the lumen of an anomalous *left* course vena cava

8.3 Metallic Stents

Endoprosthetic stents composed of metals and other materials were originally designed for intravascular use, but they have found extensive application in many other situations [15–17]. With respect to the vascular tree, they are used to maintain or restore the patency in compromised arterial and venous lumens. Angioplasty and stenting of femoral, iliac, renal, and coronary arterial lesions are common, and endovascular stents are being applied to the treatment of aortic aneurysms.

Well-known complications of these stents include intimal dissection, thrombosis, malpositioning, infections, and rupture (Fig. 8.3).

8.4 Endovascular Abdominal Aortic Aneurysm Repair

Endovascular repair of an abdominal aortic aneurysm (EVAR) was first performed by Dr Juan Parodi in Argentina in 1991 [18]. It has since gained increasing acceptance over open repair due to its low invasiveness and feasibility for high-risk patients.

Fig. 8.3 MDCT –VR reformatted image demonstrates a *left* iliac stent rupture (*arrow*)

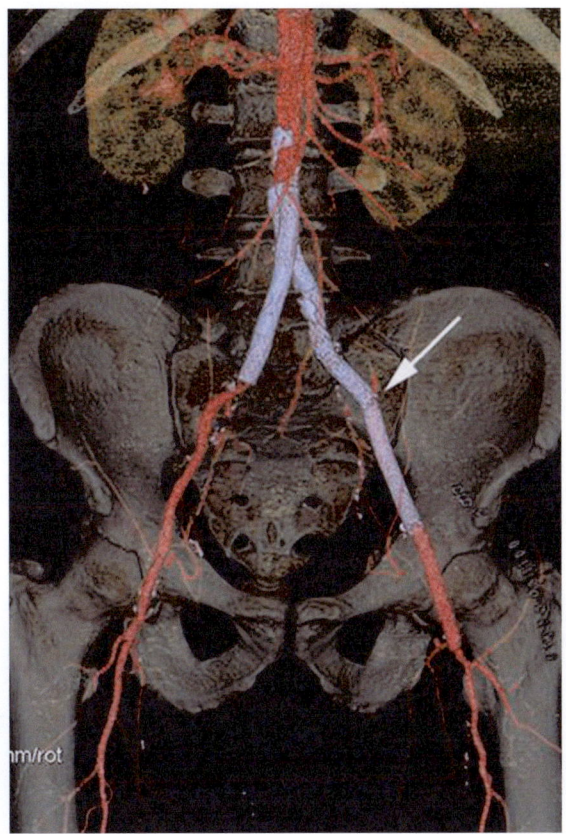

Imaging surveillance post-EVAR is accepted as mandatory to identify several complications: stent or hook fractures (Fig. 8.4), endoleaks (Fig. 8.4), separation of modular components, aneurysm enlargement, and distal migration of the endograft [19]. Moreover, any implanted device may become infected, and there are uncommon cases of infection of stent-grafts (Fig. 8.5). The appearances are similar to infected surgical grafts with retroperitoneal inflammatory change, gas in the sac, and periaortic fluid collections.

Imaging surveillance post-EVAR commonly involves Multidetector row Computed Tomography Angiography (MDCTA), which is seen as the reference standard for detection of endoleaks. This is often used in conjunction with plain radiographic films to assess device fracture, migration, or distortion. Moreover, ultrasound surveillance post-EVAR is safe and can be initiated early based on selection criteria of sac shrinkage or a stable size for 2 years; a recent meta-analysis showed the sensitivity of unenhanced ultrasound to be 0.77, although there was a promising role for contrast-enhanced ultrasound, which showed excellent sensitivity for endoleak (0.98) [20].

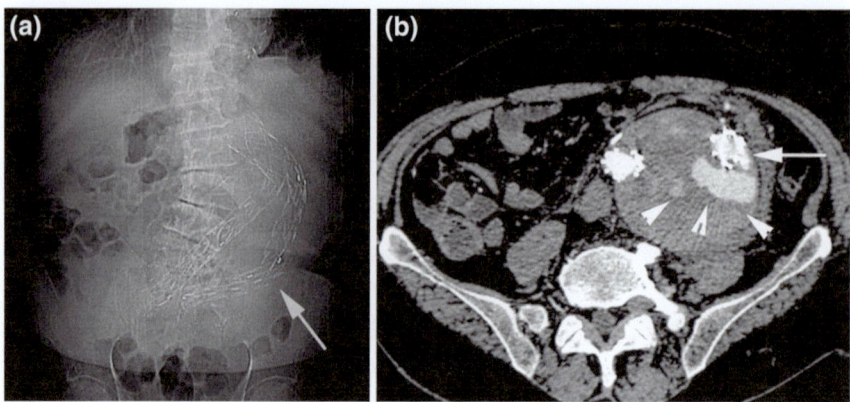

Fig. 8.4 Plain abdominal film **a** performed in patient post-EVAR shows an alteration of device configuration with *left* iliac branch rupture (*white arrow*). MDCT axial image **b** confirms the stent wire fracture (*arrow*), associated with contrast medium extravasation inside the native aortic aneurysm lumen (*arrowheads*)

Fig. 8.5 MDCT coronal reformatted image shows the infection of the aortobisiliac endoprosthesis with thrombotic lumen mixed to air bubbles (*arrows*)

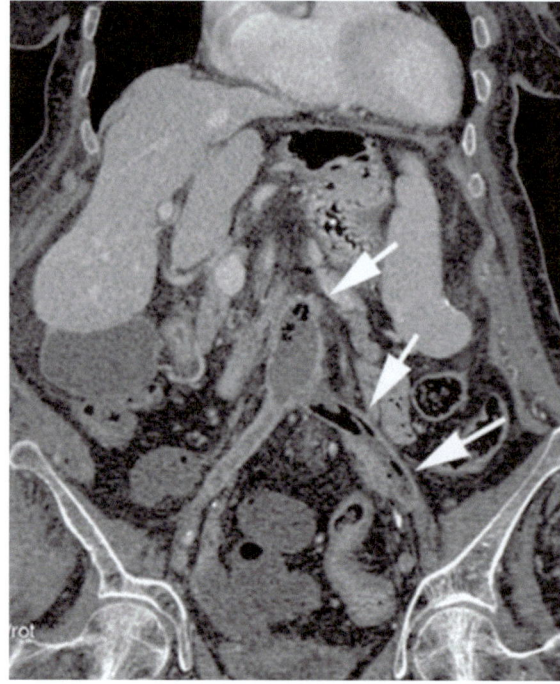

Many factors that affect the success and failure of EVAR are strongly influenced by preprocedural planning, the experience of the operator, the technique employed, and the type and the generation of the endograft.

8.5 Conclusions

It is strongly recommended that scout views for chest, abdominal, and pelvic MDCT studies be carefully examined for vascular devices. Intravascular devices fragments can cause life-threatening complications: a correct diagnosis is mandatory. Moreover, successful retrieval of these fragments can obviate the need for major surgeries.

References

1. Tan PL, Gibson M (2006) Central venous catheters: the role of radiology. Clin Radiol 61:13–22
2. Macdonald S, Watt AJ, McNally D et al (2000) Comparison of technical success and outcome of tunneled catheters inserted via the jugular and subclavian approaches. J Vasc Interv Radiol 11:225–231
3. Tseng M, Sadler D, Wong J et al (2001) Radiological placement of central venous catheters: rates of success and immediate complications in 3412 cases. Can Assoc Radiol J 52:379–384
4. Lund GB, Trerotola SO, Scheel PF Jr et al (1996) Outcome of tunneled hemodialysis catheters placed by radiologists. Radiology 198:467–472
5. Tyburski JG, Joseph AL, Thomas GA et al (1993) Delayed pneumothorax after central venous access: a potential hazard. Am Surg 59:587–589
6. Robinson JF, Robinson WA, Cohn A et al (1995) Perforation of the great vessels during central venous line placement. Arch Intern Med 155:1225–1228
7. Collier PE, Blocker SH, Graff DM et al (1998) Cardiac tamponade from central venous catheters. Am J Surg 176:212–214
8. Oliver WC Jr, Nuttall GA, Beynen FM et al (1997) The incidence of artery puncture with central venous cannulation using a modified technique for detection and prevention of arterial cannulation. J Cardiothorac Vasc Anesth 11:851–855
9. Suojanen JN, Brophy DP, Nasser I (2000) Thrombus on indwelling central venous catheters: the histopathology of "fibrin sheaths". Cardiovasc Intervent Radiol 23:194–197
10. Hoch JR (1997) Management of the complications of long-term venous access. Semin Vasc Surg 10:135–143
11. Timsit JF, Farkas JC, Boyer JM et al (1998) Central vein catheter-related thrombosis in intensive care patients: incidence, risks factors, and relationship with catheter-related sepsis. Chest 114:207–213
12. Puel V, Caudry M, Le Metayer P et al (1993) Superior vena cava thrombosis related to catheter malposition in cancer chemotherapy given through implanted ports. Cancer 72:2248–2252
13. Cadman A, Lawrance JA, Fitzsimmons L et al (2004) To clot or not to clot? That is the question in central venous catheters. Clin Radiol 59:349–355
14. Nayeemuddin M, Pherwani AD, Asquith JR (2013) Imaging and management of complications of central venous catheters. Clin Radiol 68:529–544
15. Ray CD (1981) Electrical and chemical stimulation of the CNS by direct means for pain control: present and future. Clin Neurosurg 28:564–588
16. Richardson RR, Siqueira EB, Cerullo LJ (1979) Spinal epidural neuro stimulation for treatment of acute and chronic intractable pain: initial and long term results. Neurosurgery 5:344–348
17. Jung G, Song H, Kang S et al (2000) Malignant gastroduodenal obstructions: treatment by means of a covered expandable metallic stent: intial experience. Radiology 216:758–763

18. Parodi JC, Palmaz JC, Barone HD (1991) Transfemoral intraluminal graft implantation for abdominal aortic aneurysms. Ann Vasc Surg 5:491–499
19. Fulton JJ, Farber MA, Sanchez LA et al (2006) Effect of challenging neck anatomy on midterm migration rates in AneuRx endografts. J Vasc Surg 44:932–937
20. Mirza TA, Karthikesalingam A, Jackson D et al (2010) Duplex ultrasound and contrast-enhanced ultrasound versus computed tomography for the detection of endoleak after EVAR: systematic review and bivariate meta-analysis. Eur J Vasc Endovasc Surg 39:418–428

Retained Intracranial and Intraspinal Foreign Bodies

Gianluigi Guarnieri, Luigi Genovese and Mario Muto

9.1 Introduction

Foreign bodies are any objects originating outside the body. They frequently occur due to various accidental injuries such as traffic accidents, explosions or bursts, and gunshot injuries in the maxillofacial, cranial, and spinal regions or due to spinal or cranial treatment. Depending on the type of trauma, the composition and location of the foreign bodies can vary considerably [1]. Metallic materials, except aluminum, and glass of all types are opaque on radiographs, so visualizing these materials is easier than nonopaque ones. Infection, inflammation, and pain are potential complications after impact of foreign bodies. Superficial foreign bodies are usually easy to remove if seen. Key factors influencing patient management including the type of object, its physical characteristics, the location of the object, associated medical conditions, the presence or absence of symptoms, and evidence of complications.

Penetrating foreign bodies are more difficult to remove. It is necessary to determine whether the foreign body is near a vital structure or not. The most common retained objects are wood splinters, glass fragments, and metallic objects. Localizing and retrieving foreign bodies can be complicated. Conventional plain radiographs, multidetector row computed tomography (MDCT), and magnetic resonance imaging (MRI) can be used to identify foreign bodies located at the level of the cranial or the spinal regions. MDCT is a standard method for imaging and localizing foreign bodies because their shape and size are accurately reproduced. It also enables the exact localization of a foreign body in the patient's body as a prerequisite to being removed surgically [2]. However, metallic artefacts are an important source of error when detecting foreign bodies with MDCT imaging.

9.2   Retained Intracranial Foreign Bodies

Traumatic head and brain injuries, including penetrating head injuries, are the leading cause of morbidity and mortality in young people [3, 4]. However, in some patients, these head injuries do not affect neurological function, even if the foreign body is retained in the brain parenchyma [4–6].

Penetrating injuries of the brain are very common in warfare injuries but are rarer in civilian head injuries. Missile injuries account for the majority of penetrating wounds of the brain [7] although the brain has been penetrated by almost every conceivable object. There are reports in the literature ranging from a knife [8] to blades, spoons, and even nails [9] (Fig. 9.1a–d).

The major determinant of injury is the behavior of the penetrating object within the tissue which in turn depends on deformation, yaw (rotation about the long axis), and fragmentation of the projectile. The velocity of the penetrating object has been emphasized in previous studies and differentiates wounds into "low velocity" and "high velocity." However, velocity is not an independent primary determinant of wounding potential [10].

The three most common types of low velocity penetrating head injuries are industrial accidents, suicide attempts, and results of criminal assault. Immediate radiological examination is mandatory because the small entrance wound does not correspond with the size of foreign body and associated intracranial injury. X-ray skull is useful to delineate the depth and direction of penetration.

In the civilian population, most gunshot wounds are the result of a semi-jacketed missile, which has an exposed, easily deformed, soft metal, or hollow-point tip. When deformation occurs, the diameter of the projectile may increase to two to three times its original size. The permanent cavity arises from the cutting action of the projectile and is comparable in size to the final diameter of the bullet.

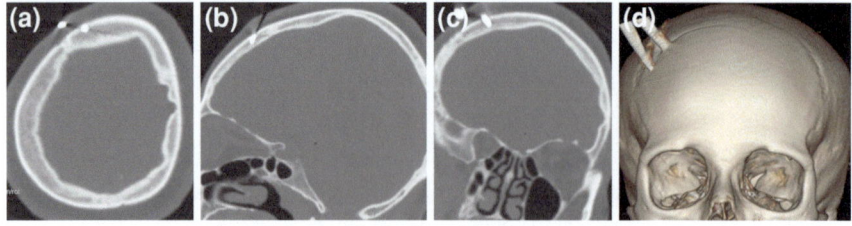

Fig. 9.1 An axial CT with bone window (**a**) and sagittal (**b**) and coronal (**c**) MPR with bone windows show a retained foreign body (a scep) into the right frontal squamous, confirmed by 3D reconstruction (**d**)

The increase in contact area also results in rapid deceleration of the missile and the release of energy into the surrounding tissues, producing a larger temporary cavity as well. Radial forces and subsequent pressure waves from the transfer of kinetic energy contribute to further tissue damage by the formation of this temporary cavity parallel to the bullet tract. The brain is extremely susceptible to the formation of both permanent and temporary cavitation [11]. The impact velocity of a missile and the incident angle influence whether the missile will penetrate the calvarium and the severity of fracture [11]. If the incident angle is small, a tangential wound may occur; that is, the missile penetrates the superficial soft tissues but does not enter the calvarium. In these wounds, the missile imparts a relatively small amount of its kinetic energy to the tissue, and the vast majority of the energy is retained by the projectile so that flight beyond the target is maintained. However, intracranial damage can occur owing to energy waves transmitted through the skull to the brain [12]. Skull fractures result when the tensile force caused by the missile exceeds the elastic properties of the skull.

Bone and bullet fragments deep within the brain parenchyma are potential sources of infection: insufficient heat is generated when firing a gun to sterilize a bullet. The necrotic tissue also provides an excellent culture medium for the growth of microorganisms, and the injured area is often lined by foreign material (hair, skin, and cloth) brought into the wound by the bullet [11]. For these reasons—secondary infection, brain edema, and hematomas can result in a fatal clinical course and death with medicolegal consequences [8]—one of the goals of the neurosurgeon is to remove all accessible bone, bullet fragments, and devitalized brain tissue [12].

In the emergency setting, when penetrating cranial injury is suspected, MDCT is considered the primary diagnostic examination [13, 14]. While MDCT easily detects metallic objects, wooden foreign bodies may be problematic in radiologic diagnosis [13]. Intracranial wood may show varying degrees of attenuation on CT scans. Dry wood, which often displays low attenuation, resembling air bubbles, should not be dismissed as air or an artifact. In subacute and chronic stages, a wooden foreign body absorbs water and approaches tissue density [13]. Although both CT and MRI imaging may be available for the detection of nonmetallic foreign bodies, such as wood and plastic, CT at various window widths should be considered the primary diagnostic technique, because MRI imaging may not differentiate dry wood from air or bone fragments [15].

In the emergency acute fashion, the CT patterns to reach on CT scan in emergency situation are:
- the presence of retained foreign bodies for example gunshot, with its hole access or exit, if not retained
- penumoencephalus
- the correlated fractures and bone fragments migration
- the parenchyma alterations correlated such as lacerocontusion, hemorrhagic intraparenchimal, or extraparenchimal collections (Epidural or Subdural hematoma, intraparenchimal satellite hematoma)
- post-traumatic Subarachnoid Hemorrhage (SAH).

- cerebral oedema
- diffuse brain damage,
- brainstem injury,
- CNS infection, or ventricular injury.

Obviously, the more of these elements that are present, the worse the patient outcomes are. [16] (Figs. 9.2a–h, 9.3a–i).

During the follow-up, an infection element such as abscess, empyema, CSF injury, must be reached.

Brain swelling and CSF leak, orbit-cranial trajectory and intraventricular lodgement are associated with increased incidence of such complications.

Patients with retained intracranial missile fragments should be on regular follow-up so that such complications are recognized and treated as they occur [17, 18].

A good practice suggests that every patient with an open wound be inspected carefully—a claim that should be self-evident. If there is any risk of existing penetrating or depressed skull trauma, CT imaging should be performed, even in patients with a Glasgow Coma Scale sum score of 14 or 15 [19, 20].

Previous studies have demonstrated that in up to 14 % of patients with a Glasgow Coma Scale of 14, CT scans showed intracranial lesions. Additional CT angiography should be performed in penetrating injuries with hematomas or suspected vascular lesions [21].

It is recommended not to perform an MRI study if a retained foreign body is present, because of uncertain foreign body nature.

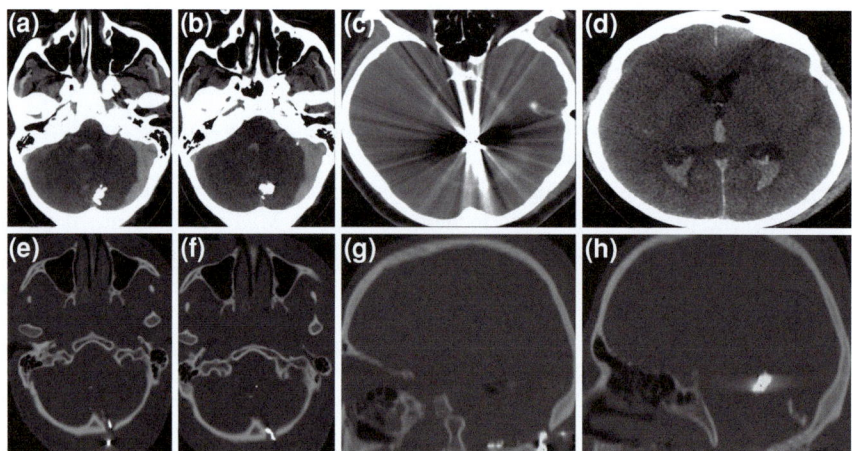

Fig. 9.2 The axial CT scan shows (**a–d**) multiple retained bullets in the posterior fossa with left subdural cerebellum haematoma and tetraventricular haematoma. The axial (**e–f**) and sagittal MPR (**g–h**) show the inlet hole at the occitial squamous and the retained bullets in the posterior fossa

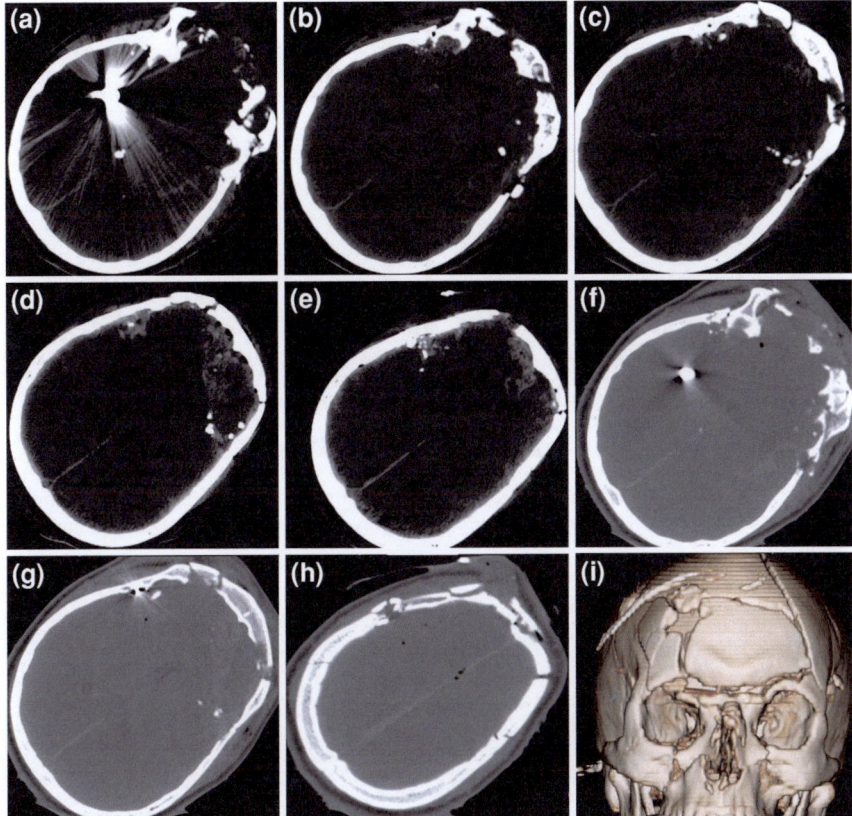

Fig. 9.3 The axial CT scan shows (**a–e**) retained bullets in the right temporal lobe with multiple fragments in the left frontal and temporal lobe. A traumatic diffuse SAH and a multiple hemorraghic left frontal contusions are present with small frontal penumoencefalus. The axial CT scan with bone window (**f–h**) shows the inlet hole a temporal squamous with retained bullet and multiple skull-bone fractures confirmed by 3D reconstruction (**i**)

All the devices used during neurointerventional procedures such as cerebral aneurism embolization, vessel stenting, AVM embolization are compatible with MRI and it can be performed without any problem and without waiting time after the procedure. The presence of these devices is easy to reach and to identify and they produce an X-ray and MRI artifacts.

As endovascular procedure complication, a retained coils migration or a retained microcatheter fragment or small metallic splinter into SAH space are described and generally they are not correlated with any type of cerebral injury or infection [22] (Fig. 9.4a, b).

In case of a retained microcatheter fragment is incorporated into the arterial wall of intracranial vessel while other portions may remain mobile and cause late peripheral arterial symptoms it should be surgically removed [23].

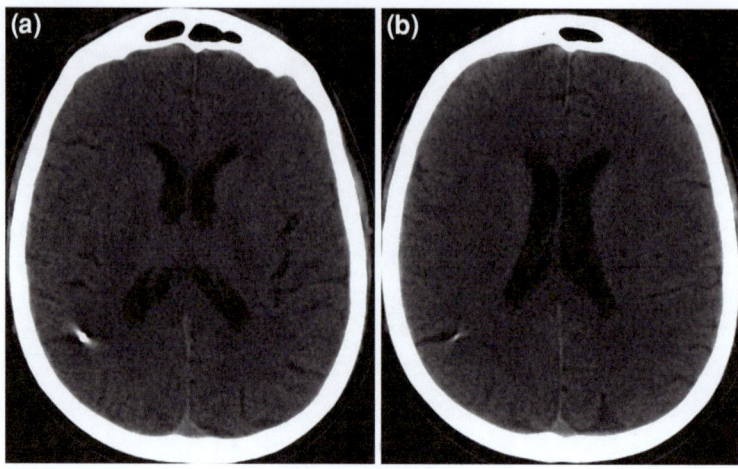

Fig. 9.4 a–b The axial CT scan shows a small retained metallic fragment in the right frontal subaracnoid space without any parenchima alteration, injected during a cerebral aneurysm embolization

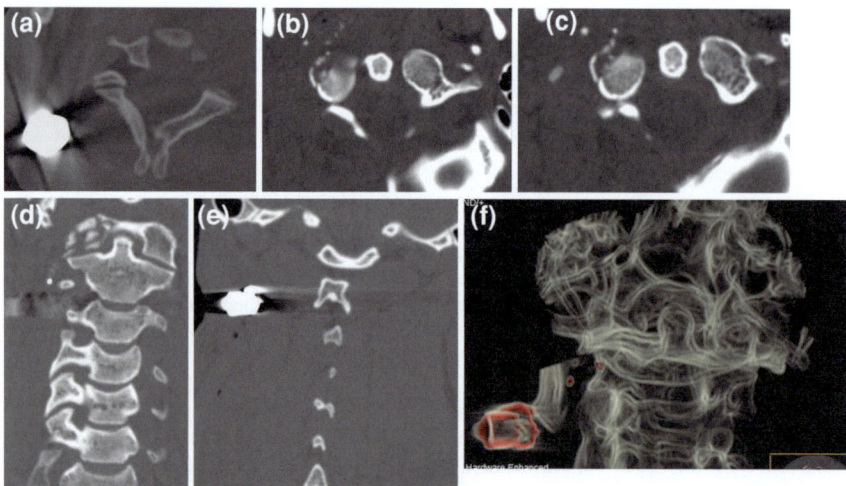

Fig. 9.5 The axial CT scan (**a**) and the Coronal MPR (**d**, **e**) and 3D-VR (**f**) show a retained bullet in the right paravertebral soft tissue with right lateral mass fracture of C1 (**b**, **c**)

9.3 Retained Intraspinal Foreign Bodies

Penetrating injuries to the spine, although less common than blunt trauma from motor vehicle accidents, are important causes of injury to the spinal cord [24, 25]. They are essentially of two varieties—gunshot or stab wounds. Gunshot injuries to

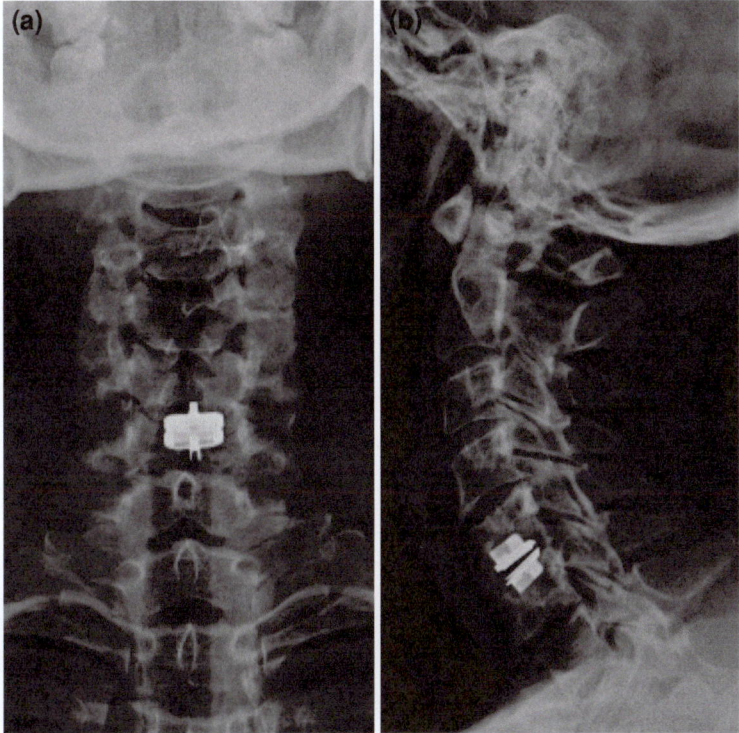

Fig. 9.6 The PA (**a**) and LL (**b**) X-ray films show an intradiscal "cage" at level C5–C6

the spine are more commonly described and are associated with a higher incidence of neurological damage. On the contrary, the prognosis is better in stab wounds where surgery plays a greater role [26].

Approximately one-third of penetrating gunshot wounds causing spinal cord injuries are likely to involve a retained bullet fragment within the spinal canal [27]. Retained canal fragments may have a more subtle clinical presentation than complete spinal transection, ranging from occult to partial cord syndromes. Although rare, retained canal fragments must always be considered in penetrating trauma. Retained canal fragments that are blunt (e.g., a bullet fragment) are recommended for surgical removal if progressive neurological symptoms develop, historically, if made of copper or lead causing toxicity and, commonly, if located below the T12 spinal level because of the risk of fragment migration [27]. Sharp retained canal fragments (e.g., a knife tip) are recommended for surgical removal irrespective of spinal level to prevent worsening of the spinal cord injury [27, 28]; moreover, it is important to be aware that if a foreign body located in the spinal canal is not surgically removed, any unexplained change in neurological symptoms or signs must be investigated immediately and surgical removal needs to be considered.

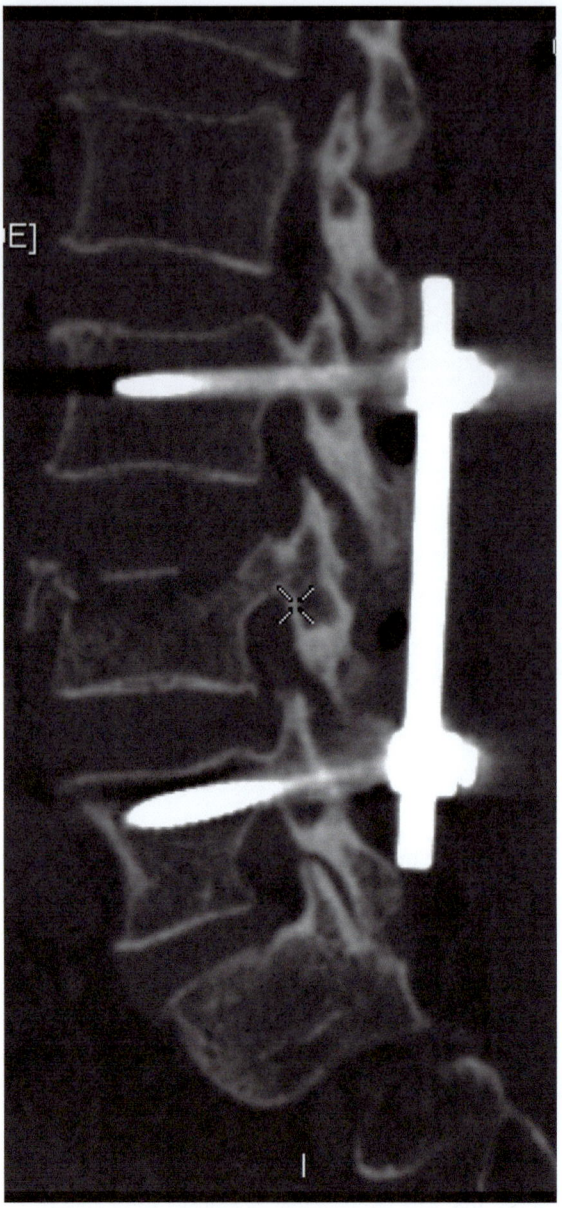

Fig. 9.7 The sagittal MPR-CT shows the good position the tranpeduncolar screws and rods at L3 and L5 levels. Somatic fracture of L4

Intraspianal migration of bullet fragments, though rare, should be included as one of the delayed complications of gunshot wound to the head [29].

It is argued that with regard to a retained bullet in the vicinity of the spinal canal, the presence or absence of neurological symptoms should be the guide for further diagnostic procedures. Only if a neurological deficit develops, which is possible after many years, should surgical intervention be considered, depending on the severity and type of the deficit [30].

Long-term retained intraspinal foreign body produces a chronic inflammation caused by metal breakdown products of the bullet contributing to the increasing back pain or neurogenic claudication and radiculopathy. It is pointed out that it is necessary to take account the kind of metal when deciding for or against the removal of a foreign body. Reaction to foreign body corrosion is believed to be the major cause of delayed neurological deficit. In this case, radiological investigations are requested to rule out morphological changes as the origin of the increase in pain [31–33].

Because of retained foreign bodies can be metallic, patients could not undergo to MRI and in acute emergency fashion or follow-up and only a MDCT scan with multiplanar and 3D reconstruction can be performed in order to reach its position, a spinal cord injury, an epidural-subdural hemorrhagic collection, or vertebral fracture (Fig. 9.5).

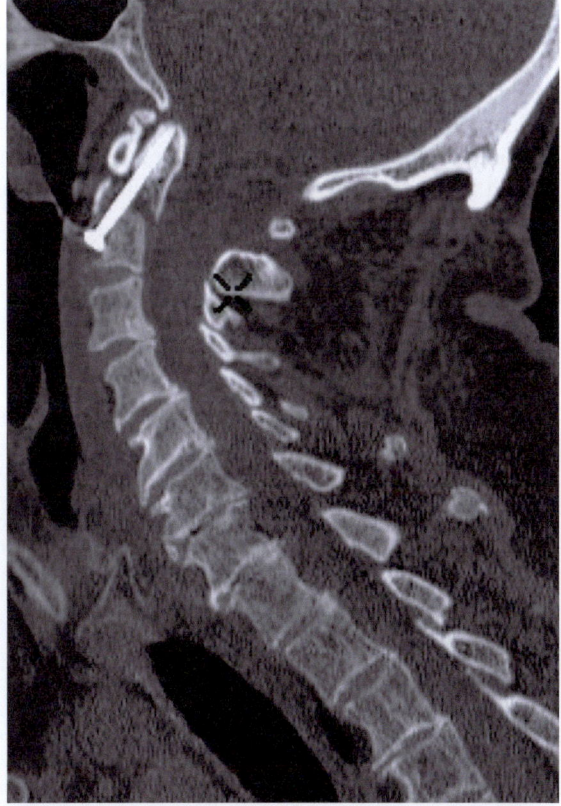

Fig. 9.8 The sagittal MPR-CT shows the good position the screw of C2

During the follow-up, the first complication of foreign body is the risk of infection. If the foreign body cannot be removed, only a CT scan with contrast element can be performed in order to exclude a empyema or infection collection.

As well as for cerebral endovascular procedure, all the devices used for interventional or surgical spinal procedures are compatible with MRI and they can be investigated by MRI and MDCT, obviously, and sometimes they can migraine into spinal canal. These devices are easy to reach and to identify and because they produce an x-ray or MRI artifacts, a CT scan should be preferred to check their right position (Figs. 9.6, 9.7, 9.8), while MRI scan should be considered to check spinal cord myelopathy or clinical worsening.

9.4 Conclusions

Radiologic assessment of penetrating cranial or spinal injuries and possible resultant foreign bodies can include plain films, CT, and MRI. Plain films are limited in their ability to delineate soft tissue and precisely localize radiopaque foreign bodies with respect to their intracranial or intraspinal location. This often necessitates a MDCT examination, which facilitates localization and better demonstrate other injuries such as cellulitis, fractures, and hemorrhage. While MDCT has much greater sensitivity than plain films in detecting foreign bodies, it may fail to detect wood fragments, as wood and air can have a similar hypoattenuative CT appearance. The MRI study to detect penetrating cranial or spinal injuries may be limited or contraindicated by the metallic and/or ferromagnetic properties of the foreign body.

References

1. Eggers G, Welzel T, Mukhamadiev D et al (2007) X-ray-based volumetric imaging of foreign bodies: a comparison of computed tomography and digital volume tomography. J Oral Maxillofac Surg 65:1880–1885
2. Eggers G, Mukhamadiev D, Hassfeld S (2005) Detection of foreign bodies of the head with digital volume tomography. Dentomaxillofac Radiol 34:74–79
3. Turbin RE, Maxwell DN, Langer PD et al (2006) Patterns of transorbital intracranial injury: a review and comparison of occult and non-occult cases. Surv Ophthalmol 51:449–460
4. Youssef AS, Morgan JM, Padhya T et al (2008) Penetrating craniofacial injury inflicted by a knife. J Trauma 64:1622–1624
5. Bhootra BL (2007) Retained intra cranial blade—medicolegal perspectives. J Forensic Leg Med 14:31–34
6. Taylor AG, Peter JC (1997) Patients with retained transcranial knife blades: a high-risk group. J Neurosurg 87:512–515
7. Kaufman HH (1991) Treatment of civilian gunshot wounds to the head. Neurosurg Clin North Am 2:387–397
8. Davis NL, Kahana T, Hiss J (2004) Souvenir knife: a retained transcranial knife blade. Am J Forensic Med Pathol 25:259–261

9. Salar G, Costella GB, Mottaran R et al (2004) Multiple craniocerebral injuries from penetrating nails. J Neurosurg 100:963
10. Fackler ML (1988) Wound ballistics. A review of common misconceptions. JAMA 259:2730–2736
11. Ragsdale BD (1984) Gunshot wounds: a historical perspective. Milit Med 149:301–315
12. Stone JA, Slone HW, Yu JS et al (1977) Gunshot wounds of the brain: influence of ballistics and predictors of outcome by computed tomography. Emerg Radiol 4:140–149
13. Hansen JE, Gudeman SK, Holgate RC et al (1988) Penetrating intracranial wood wounds: clinical limitations of computerized tomography. J Neurosurg 68:752–756
14. Etherington RJ, Hourihan MD (1989) Localisation of intraocular and intraorbital foreign bodies using computed tomography. Clin Radiol 40:610–614
15. McGuckin JF, Akhtar N Jr, Ho VT et al (1996) CT and MR evaluation of a wooden foreign body in an in vitro model of the orbit. Am J Neuroradiol 17:129–133
16. Coşar A, Gönül E, Kurt E, Gönül M, Taşar M, Yetişer S (2005) Craniocerebral gunshot wounds: results of less aggressive surgery and complications. Minim Invasive Neurosurg 48(2):113–118
17. Bhatoe HS (2001) Retained intracranial splinters: a follow up study in survivors of low intensity military conflicts. Neurol India 49(1):29–32
18. Splavski B, Sisljagić V, Perić L, Vranković D, Ebling Z (2000) Intracranial infection as a common complication following war missile skull base injury. Injury 31(4):233–237
19. Fischer BR, Yasin Y, Holling M, Hesselmann V (2012) Good clinical practice in dubious head trauma—the problem of retained intracranial foreign bodies. Int J Gen Med 5:899–902
20. Teasdale G, Jennett B (1974) Assessment of coma and impaired consciousness. A practical scale. Lancet 2(7872):81–84
21. Maas AI, Stocchetti N, Bullock R (2008) Moderate and severe traumatic Brain injury in adults. Lancet Neurol 7(8):728–741
22. Teksam M, McKinney A, Truwit CL (2004) A retained neurointerventional microcatheter fragment in the anterior communicating artery aneurysm in multi-slice computed tomography angiography. Acta Radiol 45(3):340–343
23. Zoarski GH, Lilly MP, Sperling JS, Mathis JM (1999) Surgically confirmed incorporation of a chronically retained neurointerventional microcatheter in the carotid artery. AJNR Am J Neuroradiol 20(1):177–178
24. Baghai P, Sheptak PE (1982) Penetrating spinal injury by a glass fragment: case report and review. Neurosurgery 11:419–422
25. Cybulski GR, Stone JL, Kant R (1989) Outcome of laminectomy for civilian gunshot injuries of the terminal spinal cord and cauda equina: review of 88 cases. Neurosurgery 24:392–397
26. Steinmetz MP, Krishnaney AA et al (2004) Penetrating spinal injuries. Neurosurg Q 14:217–223
27. Waters RL, Sie IH (2003) Spinal cord injuries from gunshot wounds to the spine. Clin Orthop Relat Res 408:120–125
28. Williams DT, Chang DL, DeClerck MP (2009) Penetrating spinal cord injuries with retained canal fragments. CJEM 11:172–173
29. Young WF Jr, Katz MR, Rosenwasser RH (1993) Spontaneous migration of an intracranial bullet into the cervical canal. South Med J 86(5):557–559
30. Kuijlen JM, Herpers MJ, Beuls EA (1997) Neurogenic claudication, a delayed complication of a retained bullet. Spine (Phila Pa 1976) 22(8):910–914
31. Doll M, Baum H (1989) Retained intraspinal bullet—an illustrative case report. Neurosurg Rev 12(1):67–70
32. Ajmal S, Enam SA, Shamim MS (2009) Neurogenic claudication and radiculopathy as delayed presentations of retained spinal bullet. Spine J 9(10):e5–e8
33. Fung CF, Ng TH (1992) Delayed myelopathy after a stab wound with a retained intraspinal foreign body: case report. J Trauma 32(4):539–541

Role of Magnetic Resonance Imaging in Diagnosing Foreign Bodies

10

Rosaria De Ritis, Francesco Di Pietto and Carlo Cavaliere

10.1 Foreign Bodies

Foreign body inside soft tissues is an object under skin, within muscle or fat which should not be present there normally [1]. Patients often forget and cannot always recall the memory of penetration by a foreign body. Some foreign bodies like multiple shotgun pellets do not need removal if not causing any problem. Therefore, the clinical history may be useful in narrowing the differential diagnosis in many patients.

Common foreign bodies are pieces of metal, glass, plant thorn, bamboo-stick, gravel, etc. Radio-opaque foreign bodies like metal, gravel, glass, etc., can be seen on radiographs but determining the location of radiolucent foreign bodies like wood, thorn, bamboo-sticks, etc., deep inside tissues, remaining undetected most frequently [2, 3]. A study by Anderson et al. reveals that most common foreign bodies in order of frequency are wood, glass and metal fragments. The study also shows that radiographs correctly identified metallic fragments in 100 % of cases but wood was correctly identified in only 15 % of cases [4]. Moreover, foreign bodies having sharp tips, move inside tissues due to muscular activities (Fig. 10.1) and organic materials like wood, with its porous consistency, may be infected and may cause local abscess formation which may result in a chronic discharging wound [5]. A foreign body nearby a joint may gradually erode tissues and may penetrate inside the joint, subsequently infected and may lead to joint destruction and even limb loss [6]. For this reason, a foreign body should be suspected in cases of recurrent or unexplained soft-tissue infections.

So, when the depth of foreign body affects the resolution of US technique, CT-scan or MRI is needed to detect radiolucent foreign body.

R. De Ritis (✉) · F. Di Pietto · C. Cavaliere
MR Body Unit, Cardarelli Hospital, Via A. Cardarelli 9, 80131, Napoli, Italy
e-mail: rosariaderitis@virgilio.it

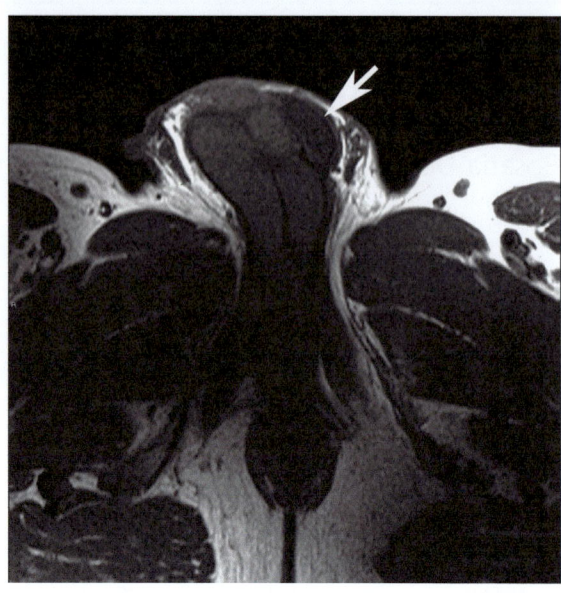

Fig. 10.1 Prosthetic device shifted inside tissues. Migration in the soft tissues of a penile prosthesis consisting of a reservoir shifted in the paravesical region, pumps in the corpus cavernosum, and storage tank in the scrotum (*arrow*)

10.2 Role of Magnetic Resonance Imaging

Signal intensity artifacts are often encountered during magnetic resonance (MR) imaging [7] (Fig. 10.2), and may be caused by a ferromagnetic foreign body in the imager: these cases are easily identified on radiographs and may limit MRI indication.

The utility of MR imaging in the localization of nonmetallic foreign bodies in the soft tissues of the body is well known [8, 9]. For many time, its high cost has precluded its routine use for evaluating all open injuries suspected of harboring nonradiopaque foreign bodies, however, the recent spread of MRI machines has re-evaluated this topic.

MRI can detect foreign bodies but it may be difficult to distinguish low signal intensity foreign bodies from tendons, scar tissue and calcified area. MRI shows the foreign bodies as low signal or signal void to the muscles on both T1- and T2-weighted images [10]. However, the identification of foreign bodies is difficult on MRI when the bodies are small.

Bodne et al. [11] commented on the absence of signal on MR images of retained foreign bodies composed of wood. Plastic material, which is inert and nonreactive, also can produce signal void on MR images. If the foreign body is long and thin, the lesion may present a "target appearance" when imaged in cross section. More often, MRI is employed to identify infective complications and to differentiate its soft-tissue masses [12, 13], where the detection of these lesions and their extent is better delineated with MRI than CT [11, 14].

Fig. 10.2 Metallic foreign body occasionally identified by MRI. Cardiac MRI documenting an artifact constant signal (*arrow*) due to a tiny metal chips at the left ventricle in an underwater fishing man hospitalized under emergency for TIA

When a foreign body is surrounded by inflammatory tissues or a hematoma, a ring of low signal on T1- and high signal on T2-weighted images around the foreign bodies is observed demonstrating a target appearance [15]. The surrounding reactive lesion is easily mistaken for a soft-tissue neoplasm when a foreign body is not identified because the peripheral area of the lesion is strongly enhanced by gadolinium [10]. The central area of the reactive lesion is observed as low intensities on T1- and high intensities on T2-weighted images with no enhancement, which suggests that the lesion is myxomatous or cystic [16, 17]. The key to diagnose correctly on MRI is identification of a low signal or signal void lesion inside the mass and the surrounding ring-like reactive lesion.

References

1. Pramanik MAK, Bhaduri J, Rashid AM et al (2007) Foreign body (bamboo splinter of broom stick) in soft tissue. J Teachers Assoc 20:67–70
2. Russel RC, Williamson DA, Sullivan JW et al (1991) Detection of foreign bodies in the hand. J Hand Surg Am 10:163–176
3. Flomm LL, Gl Ellis (1992) Radiologic evaluation of foreign bodies. Emerg Med Clin North Am 10:163–176
4. Anderson MA, Newmeyer WL, Kingore ES (1982) Diagnosis and treatment of retained foreign bodies in the hand. Am J Surg 144:63–67
5. Zenter J, Hassler W, Petersen D (1991) A wooden foreign body penetrating the superior orbital fissure. Neurochirurgia 34:188–190
6. Gooding GA, Hardiman T, Sumers M et al (1987) Sonography of the hand and foot in foreign body detection. J Ultrasound Med 6:441–447

7. Jones RW, Witte RJ (2000) Signal intensity artifacts in clinical MR imaging. RadioGraphics 20:893–901
8. LoBue TD, Deutsch TA, Lobick J et al (1988) Detection and localization of nonmetallic intraocular foreign bodies by magnetic resonance imaging. Arch Ophthalmol 106:260–326
9. Oikarinen KS, Nieminen TM, Makarainen H et al (1993) Visibility of foreign bodies in soft tissue in plain radiographs, computed tomography, magnetic resonance imaging, and ultrasound: an in vitro study. Int J Oral Maxillofac Surg 22:119–124
10. Peterson JJ, Bancroft LW, Kransdorf MJ (2002) Wooden foreign bodies: imaging appearance. Am J Roentgenol 178:557–562
11. Bodne D, Quinn SF, Cochran CF (1988) Imaging foreign glass and wooden bodies of the extremities with CT and MR. J Comput Assist Tomogr 12:608–611
12. Monu JUV, McManus CK, Wg Ward et al (1995) Soft-tissues masses caused by long-standing foreign bodies in the extremities: MR imaging findings. Am J Roentgenol 165:395–397
13. Ando A, Hatori M, Hagiwara Y et al (2009) Imaging features of foreign body granuloma in the lower extremities mimicking a soft tissue neoplasm. Upsala J Med Sci 114:46–51
14. Ho VT, McGuckin JF, Smergel EM (1996) Intraorbital wooden foreign body: CT and MR appearance. Am J Neuroradiol 17:134–136
15. Bode KS, Haggerty CJ, Krause J (2007) Latent foreign body synovitis. J Foot Ankle Surg 46:291–296
16. Chiba T, Hatori M, Abe Y et al (1998) Periosteal ganglion of the radius: a case report. Tohoku J Exp Med 185:71–78
17. Shibata T, Hatori M, Satoh T et al (2003) Magnetic resonance imaging features of epidermoid cyst in the extremities. Arch Orthop Trauma Surg 123:239–241

Soft Tissue Foreign Bodies

11

Antonio Pinto, Amelia Sparano and Mario Tecame

11.1 Introduction

Penetrating object injuries represent a common problem in the emergency department, and retained foreign body in soft tissues may complicate such injuries. A retained foreign body (FB) in the soft tissue may determine severe infection or inflammatory reaction; due to this reason, the detection and the removal of the FB is necessary [1]. Punctured wounds and soft tissue lacerations are clinically inspected, palpated, and explored to exclude the presence of FB; unfortunately, retained FB in the soft tissue can seldom be identified and removed on the basis of clinical examination alone. Imaging techniques are required to identify the FB and establish its exact location prior to surgical removal attempt. Radiographic evaluations are routinely performed in order to confirm the presence of radio-opaque FBs (Fig. 11.1) such as glass, metal, and stone within the soft tissue [2, 3].

Cheap and easy availability of conventional radiography makes it the first line investigation in any setting. Limitations of radiography include nonvisualization of radiolucent FBs, radiation exposure, and failure of precise localization during removal.

Failure to remove FBs is likely to give rise to acute or late complications, such as allergies, inflammation, or infection, that may be severe.

A. Pinto (✉) · A. Sparano
Department of Diagnostic Radiological Imaging, Cardarelli Hospital,
Via A. Cardarelli 9, 80131, Naples, Italy
e-mail: antopin1968@libero.it

A. Sparano
e-mail: ameliasparano@yahoo.it

M. Tecame
Department "Magrassi-Lanzara", Second University of Naples,
Piazza Miraglia 2, 80138, Naples, Italy

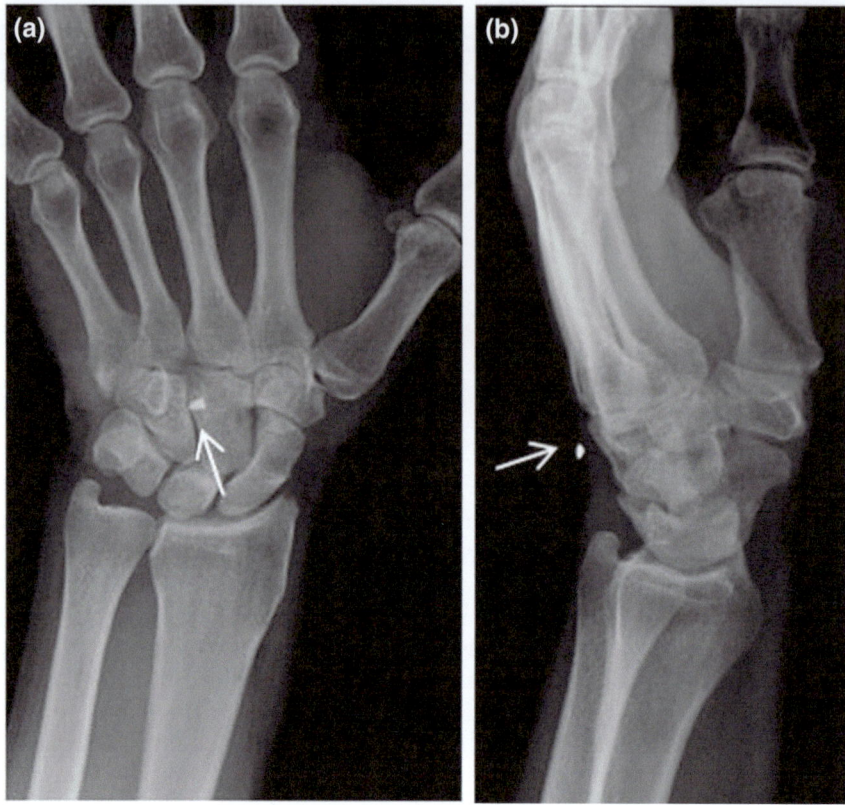

Fig. 11.1 Plain film of the carpus (two projections, **a** and **b**) shows a metallic foreign body (*arrow*) located in the soft tissues

Knowledge of the exact location of FB relative to skin surfaces, adjacent muscles, tendons, neurovascular bundles, and other vascular structures allows more controlled surgical dissection.

Soft Tissue Foreign Bodies

FBs retained in the soft tissues are a common reason for medical consultation, and usually consist of wooden or metal splinters or glass shards.

Self-inserted soft-tissue FBs, the deliberate and direct destruction or alteration of body tissue without suicidal intent, is a relatively recent focus of scrutiny by the medical community [4]. In the United States, 4 % of the general population and 13–23 % of adolescents report a history of nonsuicidal self-injury [5, 6]. These numbers are potentially underestimated as a result of underreporting due to the socially unacceptable nature of the act and the feelings of guilt experienced by the patient after the self-injury [5, 7].

11 Soft Tissue Foreign Bodies

Most metallic materials are opaque on radiographs. However, some referring physicians do not realize that thorns, splinters, wooden fragments, and pieces of plastic are usually not sufficiently opaque to be visualized [8–12]. On the other hand, glass of all types is radio-opaque [8, 9, 13]. The opacity of glass is not related to its lead content; therefore, all substantially large pieces of glass should be visible on radiographs.

Bullet wounds are far too common in the United States. Bullets (Fig. 11.2) are usually described by their caliber, which is a measurement of their diameter in inches or in millimeters. Although the caliber of a bullet is important, it has only a loose relationship to the weight of the bullet and the size of its charge. These latter parameters help determine the kinetic energy of the bullet, which is an important factor in determining its wounding potential. Bullets are usually composed of lead, and they may be fully or partially covered by an outer metal jacket (full metal jacket) that is usually composed of copper.

Bullet injuries are most severe in friable solid organs (e.g., the liver and brain), where damage may be caused by temporary cavitation remote from the actual bullet track. Dense tissues (e.g., bone) and loose tissues (e.g., subcutaneous fat) are more resistant to bullet injury. Bones modify the behavior of bullets markedly, altering their course, slowing them down, and increasing their deformity and fragmentation [14].

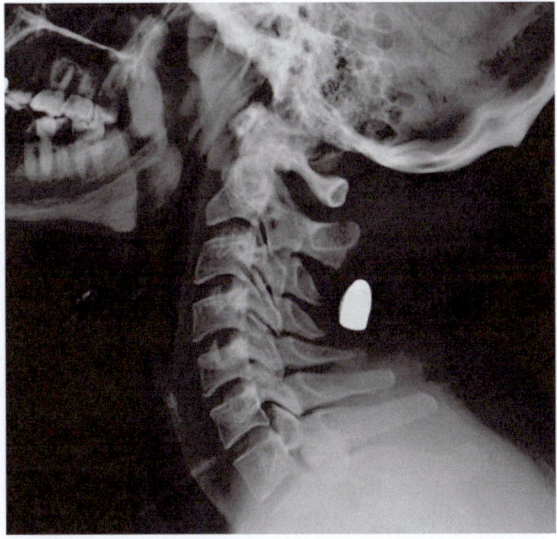

Fig. 11.2 Lateral radiograph of the neck shows the presence of a projectile lodged in the soft tissues posteriorly to the spinous process of C3–C4

Role of Imaging Procedures in the Detection of Soft Tissue Foreign Bodies

FBs can seldom be identified and removed on the basis of clinical examination alone, and usually only when superficially located at the level of the soft tissues. Otherwise, imaging techniques are required to recognize the FB and establish its exact location prior to surgical removal attempt. Conventional radiography is still now the first radiological procedure performed in patients with a clinical suspicion of soft tissue FB. Two projections are required in order to best determine the location of the FB (Fig. 11.3).

Traditional radiography usually demonstrate radio-opaque FBs (Fig. 11.4); the radiological visualization of FBs depends on their radiopacity. Metal objects with a relatively high atomic weight are easily visible on plain films even if they are millimetric (Fig. 11.5). Almost all objects composed of plastic and most thin aluminum objects, such as pull tabs on cans, are not radio-opaque. Aluminum is of low radiodensity, which makes visualization on radiographs difficult [15]. The atomic numbers of soft tissue and aluminum (7.5 and 13, respectively) are similar [16].

Glass is always radio-opaque, and its radio-opacity does not depend on its content of lead or other metals. Glass FB, whether ingested, inserted into a body cavity, or deposited in the soft tissues of an extremity by an injury, should always be detectable on radiographs. This detectability obviously depends on the size of the object. Submillimeter pieces of glass buried deep in the soft tissue of an obese person may not be visible. However, any substantial piece of glass 1–2 mm or larger should generally be detected.

As traditional radiograms are widely available, simple to perform, and inexpensive, X-ray is the reference first diagnostic examination [17] and will identify radio-opaque FBs (glass, metal, stone) in around 80 % of cases, but only displays 15 % of nonradio-opaque FBs (wood, plastic) [18, 19]. Radioscopy offers a more accurate topographic assessment and allows reference points to be marked on the skin to aid subsequent FB removal. However, radioscopy exposes patient and operator alike to relatively high doses of ionizing radiation.

Ultrasonography has now proved irreplaceable, with high sensibility and specificity [17, 20–22]. Ultrasonography is the first choice investigation in the diagnosis of an FB retained in the soft tissues, as it has a sensitivity and specificity of 90 and 96 %, respectively [23, 24]. Due to its high spatial resolution, ultrasound will identify FBs smaller than a millimetre [25], be they wood, glass, metal, or plastic [26]. The limitations of ultrasound are well known; it is an operator-dependent technique and will only display FBs retained in superficial tissues [26].

Ultrasound examination will also establish the integrity of the surrounding ligaments, tendons, joint capsules, and neurovascular structures (with the aid of color Doppler) and accurately depict the relations between the FB and adjacent structures (tendons, nerves, vessels) to ensure the safe removal of the FB, avoiding iatrogenic lesions or complications [26].

Fig. 11.3 Radiographs (two projections) of a 5-year-boy who stepped on a nail show the nail (**a** and **b**, *arrow*) in the soft tissue of his foot

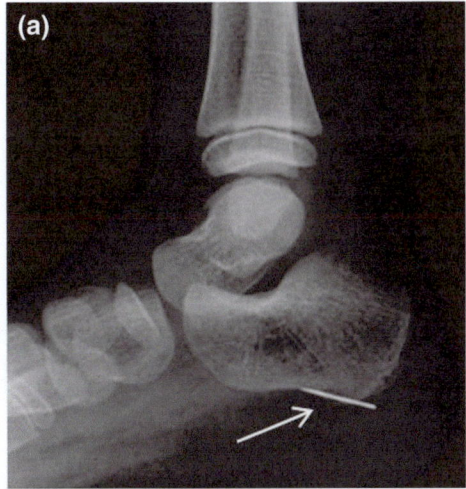
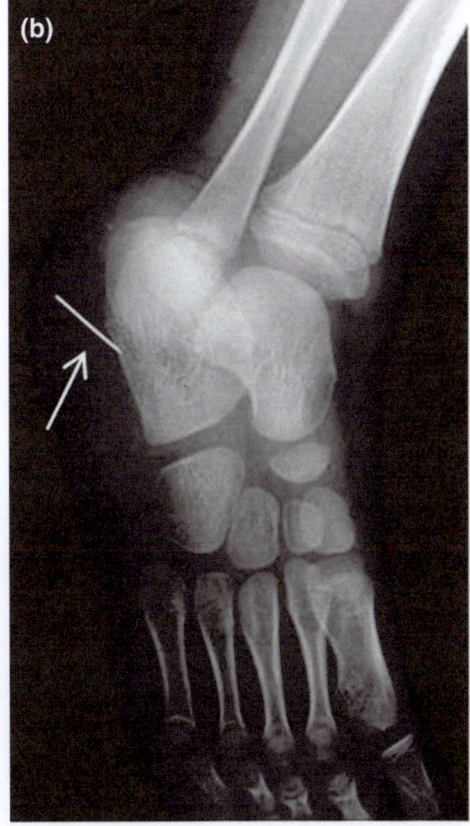

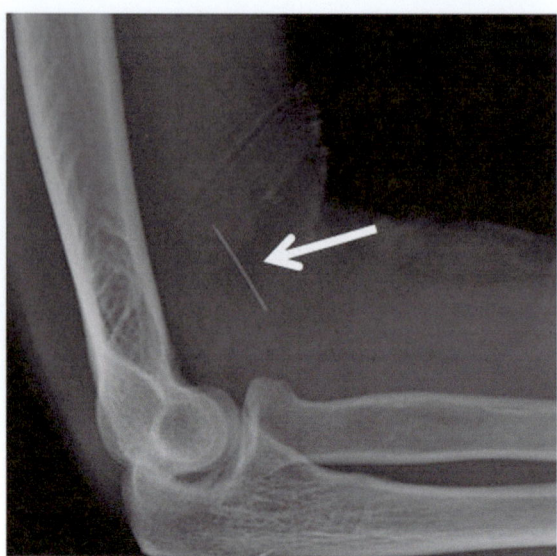

Fig. 11.4 Lateral radiograph of elbow shows the presence of a radio-opaque foreign body (*needle, arrow*) located in the soft tissues

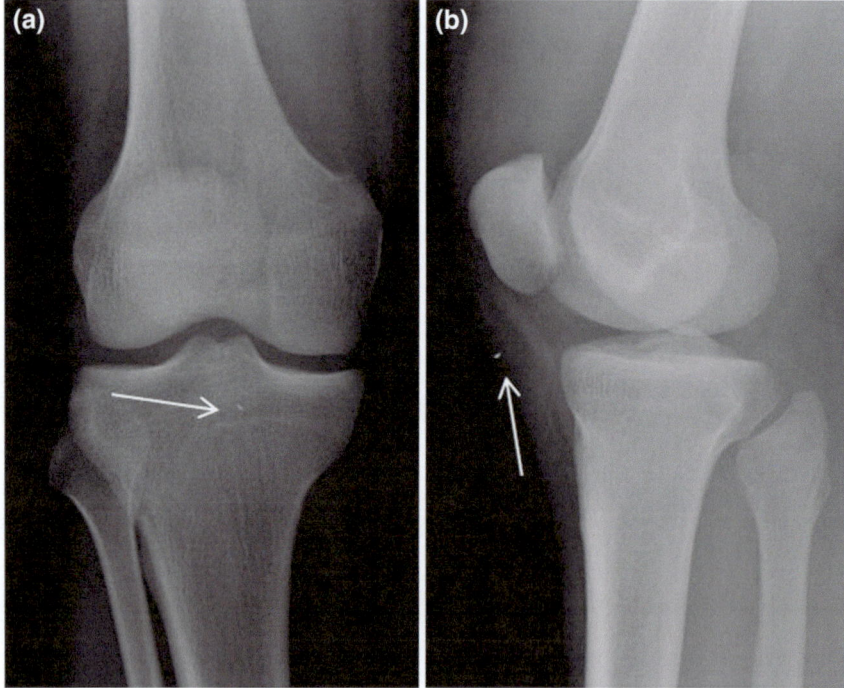

Fig. 11.5 Antero-posterior (**a**) and lateral (**b**) radiographs of the knee demonstrate the presence of a millimetric foreign body (*arrow*) located in the soft tissue region inferiorly to the rotula

Moreover, ultrasound-guided percutaneous removal of FBs is a safe and viable approach to the management of FBs achieving at least 88 % success overall [27].

Computed tomography (CT) and Magnetic Resonance (MR) scans are very expensive and have very limited indications for FB detection as they have poor sensitivity and specificity [17, 21, 24].

When compared with ultrasonography, MR is more expensive, less readily available, and has less value in the detection of small wooden FBs. Likewise, MR has obvious limitations for the evaluation of patients in the emergency room.

Complications Due to Soft Tissue Foreign Bodies

When FBs are located within or close to tendons, they may lead to irritative or septic, acute or chronic peritendinitis, or tenosynovitis. In or near a nerve, an FB may give rise to acute lesions, posttraumatic neuromas, or neuropathies [28]. FBs may also migrate to deeper soft tissues, into the joints [29–31], or even into blood vessels with possible embolic complications [32]. Long-term retention of FBs has also led to the onset of tumors [33].

Key factors influencing patient management include the type of object, its physical characteristics, the location of the object, the time elapsed since the presence of the FB in the soft tissue, the presence or absence of symptoms, and evidence of complications.

Conclusions

Even the most sheltered individual has a life filled with a multitude of minor injuries, including falls, cuts, abrasions, scratches, and burns. Everyone has suffered puncture wounds from splinters, needles, and thorns and has been cut with glass.

A retained FB in the soft tissues of extremities is not very common. Diagnosis requires high index of suspicion. Exclusion of its presence is important, given the possible allergic, inflammatory, and infectious complications associated with a retained FB. Conventional radiographs should be obtained to rule out the presence of radio-opaque foreign objects, but several types of radiolucent Fbs such as wood remain undetected on plain radiograph. Ultrasonography is the modality of choice for identification of radiolucent FBs. Ultrasound-guided percutaneous removal of FBs is a safe and viable approach to the management of FBs.

References

1. Mohamadi A, Kodabakhsh M (2010) Wooden foreign body in lung parenchyma: a case report. Turk J Trauma Emerg Surg 16:480–482
2. Flom LL, Ellis GL (1992) Radiologic evaluation of foreign bodies. Emerg Med Clin North Am 10:163–177

3. Graham DD Jr (2002) Ultrasound in the emergency department: detection of wooden foreign bodies in the soft tissues. J Emerg Med 22:75–79
4. Favazza AR (1998) The coming of age of self-mutilation. J Nerv Ment Dis 186:259–268
5. Briere J, Gil E (1998) Self-mutilation in clinical and general population samples: prevalence, correlates, and functions. Am J Orthopsychiatry 68:609–620
6. Jacobson CM, Gould M (2007) The epidemiology and phenomenology of non-suicidal self-injurious behavior among adolescents: a critical review of the literature. Arch Suicide Res 11:129–147
7. Young AS, Shiels WE 2nd, Murakami JW et al (2010) Self-embedding behavior: radiologic management of self-inserted soft-tissue foreign bodies. Radiology 257:233–239
8. Tandberg D (1982) Glass in hand and foot. Will an x-ray film show it? JAMA 248:1872–1874
9. Gordon D (1985) Non-metallic foreign bodies. Br J Radiol 58:574
10. Fornage BD, Schernberg FL (1986) Sonographic diagnosis of foreign bodies of the distal extremities. AJR Am J Roentgenol 147:567–569
11. deLacey G, Evans R, Sandin B (1985) Penetrating injuries: how easy is it to see glass (and plastic) on radiographs? Br J Radiol 58:27–30
12. Spouge AR, Weisbrod GL, Herman SJ et al (1990) Wooden foreign body in the lung parenchyma. AJR Am J Roentgenol 154:999–1001
13. Buzzard AJ, Waxman BP (1979) A long standing, much travelled rectal foreign body. Med J Aust 1:600
14. Pinto A, Brunese L, Scaglione M et al (2009) Gunshot injuries in the neck area: ballistics elements and forensic issues. Semin Ultrasound CT MRI 30:215–220
15. Conners GP (2000) Finding aluminum foreign bodies. Pediatr Rev 21:172
16. Stewart GD, Lakshmi MV, Jackson A (1994) Aluminum ring pulls: an invisible foreign body. J Accid Emerg Med 11:201–203
17. Shiels WE 2nd, Babcock DS, Wilson JL et al (1990) Localization and guided removal of soft-tissue foreign bodies with sonography. AJR Am J Roentgenol 155:1277–1281
18. Peterson JJ, Bancroft LW, Kransdorf MJ (2002) Wooden foreign bodies: imaging appearance. AJR Am J Roentgenol 178:557–562
19. Anderson MA, Newmeyer WL, Kilgore ES (1982) Diagnosis and treatment of retained foreign bodies in the hand. Am J Surg 144:63–67
20. Blankstein A, Cohen I, Heiman Z et al (2001) Ultrasonography as a diagnostic modality and therapeutic adjuvant in the management of soft tissue foreign bodies in the lower extremities. Isr Med Assoc J 3:411–413
21. Boyse TD, Fessell DP, Jacobson JA et al (2001) US of soft-tissue foreign bodies and associated complications with surgical correlation. Radiographics 21:1251–1256
22. Gibbs TS (2006) The use of sonography in the identification, localization and removal of soft tissue foreign bodies. J Diagn Med Sonogr 22:5–21
23. Jacobson JA, Powell A, Craig JG et al (1998) Wooden foreign bodies in soft tissue: detection at US. Radiology 206:45–48
24. Bray PW, Mahoney JL, Campbell JP (1995) Sensitivity and specificity of ultrasound in the diagnosis of foreign bodies in the hand. J Hand Surg Am 20:661–666
25. Ng SY, Songra AK, Bradley PF (2003) A new approach using intraoperative ultrasound imaging for localization and removal of multiple foreign bodies in the neck. Int J Oral Maxillofac Surg 32:433–436
26. Callegari L, Leonardi A, Bini A et al (2009) Ultrasound-guided removal of foreign bodies: personal experience. Eur Radiol 19:1273–1279
27. Bradley M (2012) Image-guided soft-tissue foreign body extraction. Success and pitfalls. Clin Radiol 67:531–534
28. Choudhari KA, Muthu T, Tan MH (2001) Progressive ulnar neuropathy caused by delayed migration of a foreign body. Br J Neurosurg 15:263–265
29. Gutierrez V, Radice F (2003) Late bullet migration into the knee joint. Arthroscopy 19:E15

30. Ozsunar Y, Tali ET, Kilic K (1998) Unusual migration of a foreign body from the gut to a vertebral body. Neuroradiology 40:673–674
31. Combalìa-Aleu A, Fuster-Obregon S (1993) Migration of a Kirschner wire from the sternum to the right ventricle. a case report. Am J Sports Med 21:763–764
32. Gschwind CR (2002) The intravenous foreign body: a report of 2 cases. J Hand Surg Am 27:350–354
33. Teltzrow T, Hallermann C, Muller S et al (2006) Foreign body induced angiosarcoma 60 years after a shell splinter injury. Mund Kiefer Gesichtschir 10:415–418

Foreign Bodies and Penetrating Injuries

12

Giorgio Bocchini, Giacomo Sica, Franco Guida, Luigi Palumbo, Sujit Vaida and Mariano Scaglione

12.1 Introduction

Penetrating wounds represent a wide group of life-threatening lesions to be carefully evaluated in terms of clinical context and instrumental findings.

Injuries caused by foreign bodies include a wide spectrum of lesions: from the shallow wound without a significant organ damage up to severe lacerations of parenchyma, hollow viscera, skeletal damage, in the presence or absence of actively bleeding vascular injuries that represent the most feared cause of death.

The most common causes of penetrating wounds are represented by stab and gunshot, although tissue damage can be caused by sharp metal objects, wood, glass fragments, or any other objects able to penetrate into the human body both accidentally or voluntary.

Laparotomy has always been considered the 'first line' approach in patients with gunshot wounds and penetrating injuries especially in presence of peritonitis or hemodynamic instability [1–4].

However, in the recent decades, the practice of *'non-operative management'* has significantly increased in stable patients with stab wounds and absence of clinical signs of peritoneal insult; as a result, a significant reduction of nontherapeutic or negative laparotomies have been observed, with an incidence ranging from 23 to 53 % [5]. Furthermore, also the percentage of post-operative complications has significantly decreased [4–6]. In this context, the role of imaging is of

---

S. Vaida · M. Scaglione (✉)
Department of Diagnostic Imaging, The Royal London Hospital, Whitechapel Road, London, UK
e-mail: mscaglione@tiscali.it

G. Bocchini · G. Sica · F. Guida · L. Palumbo · M. Scaglione
Department of Diagnostic Imaging, Pineta Grande Medical Center, Via Domiziana Km. 30, 81030, Castel Volturno, CE, Italy

vital importance, allowing a rapid, safe, and accurate assessment of the injuries and to direct the patient to the proper and timely management.

Particularly, Computed Tomography (CT) performed in stable and/or semi-stable patients, can exclude organ damage and actively bleeding injuries, thus avoiding unnecessary emergency laparotomies and directing the patient to conservative management. At the same time, CT examination can safely detect a wide spectrum of life-threatening injuries in a preclinical stage, i.e., before they can reach the level of clinical evidence.

Some prospective and retrospective studies conducted in the last decades have stressed the role of CT in the staging of stable patient suffering from penetrating wound of the torso [7–20]. In particular, in patients with penetrating trauma who do not require immediate surgery, they demonstrated high accuracy of the method, with sensitivity and specificity equal to 97 % [15]. However, debate still remains on gunshot wounds, in which the surgical approach is still considered essential because of the high incidence of related complications. In these cases, just a small percentage of patients is managed conservatively [15–20].

12.2 Diagnostic Approach and CT Technique

Considering the thoracoabdominal district, plain film examination can help diagnose the presence of parenchymal lung contusion, pneumothorax, pneumomediastinum, skeletal fractures, free air in the peritoneal cavity, and the presence of radiopaque foreign bodies. However, conventional radiology is not able to exclude further life-threatening injuries such as vascular lesions and/or abdominal solid organ injuries [21, 22]. In the same way, ultrasounds (US) does not provide a full and definitive assessment of penetrating torso trauma and cannot exclude most gastrointestinal and/or retroperitoneal injuries. When US is negative, the presence of hollow viscera, vessel, or diaphragmatic injuries cannot be excluded, and further diagnostic studies must be performed. On the other way, the presence of intraperitoneal free fluid alone is not an adequate parameter to indicate the need for urgent laparotomy [14, 23].

As just mentioned before, CT with intravenous contrast agent represents the 'gold standard' in this context, thus providing a full, rapid, and noninvasive patient's assessment. MDCT technique consists of a nonenhanced scan, which is useful to recognize foreign bodies, followed by a multiphasic contrastographic study with intravenous high-flow injection of contrast material (100–120 ml, rate 4–5 ml/sec). The arterial phase, acquired with the technique of 'bolus tracking', provides important diagnostic information such as the characterization of vascular injuries, whereas a portal phase (70 s from the beginning of the injection of the medium of contrast) is useful for the evaluation of parenchymas. The delayed phase is performed in selected cases, to further improve characterization of vascular injuries and/or recognize/differentiate them from injuries to the collecting system [20, 24].

In cases of suspected bladder lacerations, a full retrograde filling of the bladder with iodinated contrast agent in water solution (ratio of 1:10) is required. Identification of the site of injury is essential in terms of management, as intraperitoneal bladder injuries usually require a surgical approach whereas extraperitoneal lesions can be safely treated nonoperatively [25, 26].

In patients with penetrating thoracoabdominal injury with suspect of perforation of a hollow organ, it is also suggested the 'triple contrast CT' protocol that includes intravenous as well as orally and rectally administered contrast (1 L of a 1:25 dilution of water-soluble contrast) in order to obtain the luminal opacification of the digestive tract. It has been reported that this technique has greatly increased the accuracy of CT in the detection of traumatic perforation of the small and large intestine and represents a frequent use of technique in trauma centers, where the clinical condition of the patient permits [12–15]. However, at our institution, all initial CT scans are usually obtained without oral and/or rectal contrast. The use of CM is reserved for follow up/second look CT evaluations, just in selected cases in which bowel injuries have been previously suspected or to confirm specific findings such as extravasation from the hollow viscus lumen.

12.3 CT Findings and Indication for Treatment

At axial CT scans and Multiplanar Reformations (MPR) it is possible to recognize the "hole" of entrance as a focal defect in the skin profile, usually associated with adjacent fat stranding and subcutaneous emphysema (Fig. 12.1). The exit wound can also be determined, as well as the trajectory of the foreign body, thus providing for careful evaluation of the potentially injured organs along its course. CT also allows easy identification of foreign bodies such as bullets or fragments of any solid material. Sometimes the impact of a projectile on a osseous structure can cause its fragmentation and distribution on the adjacent tissues; in these cases, nonenhanced CT scans may be more relevant [20].

Considering the chest, penetrating traumas are associated with a high incidence of pneumothorax, hemothorax, lung contusions and lacerations and vertebrocostal fractures. When bullets or fragments get in between the vertebral bone structures, there is high risk of spinal cord injury (Fig. 12.2). Documentation of mediastinal vessels or main bronchi lesions is quite rare, since these injuries are mostly incompatible with life.

In abdominal and pelvic regions, recognition of peritoneal injuries is essential for the correct patient's management. Abdominal violation is evident when a wound is associated with hemorrhage, free air and fluid, fat stranding, bullets or

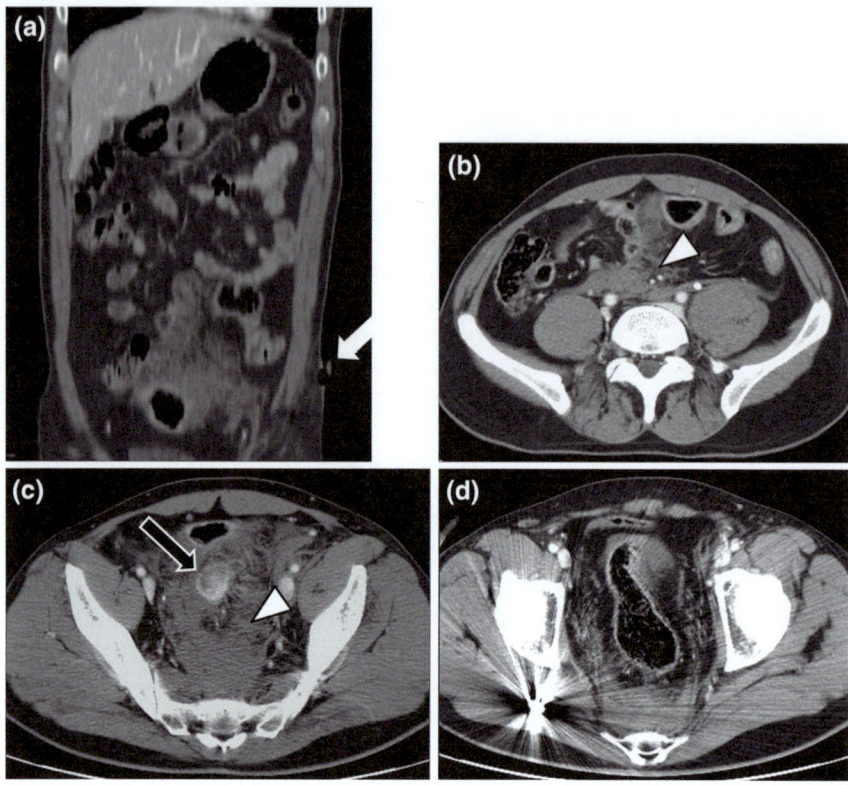

Fig. 12.1 Male, 62 years old, suffering from a gunshot wound to the left flank. **a** Coronal MPR image demonstrates the bullet entrance hole as a focal defect of the skin at the left flank associated with subcutaneous fat tissue stranding (*white arrow*). **b, c** Two noncontiguous axial scans show a hematoma at the mesenteric root (**b**, *arrowhead*) and meso-sigma (**c**, *arrowhead*) with an active bleeding pooling (**c**, *arrow*) along the course of the bullet trajectory. **d** At the end of its course, the bullet lies between the large and small gluteus muscles

any other fragment in the peritoneal cavity. Intraperitoneal free fluid or air associated or not with solid organ, hollow viscus and/or mesenteric/vascular injuries should be carefully considered because they may also come from extraperitoneal structures [15, 20].

Small and large bowel are the most frequently injured organs as a result of penetrating wounds. Extravasation of contrast medium into the extraluminal space or direct evidence of a discontinuity in the viscera wall, represent the highest specific signs of gastrointestinal transmural injury. These signs usually require an immediate surgical approach.

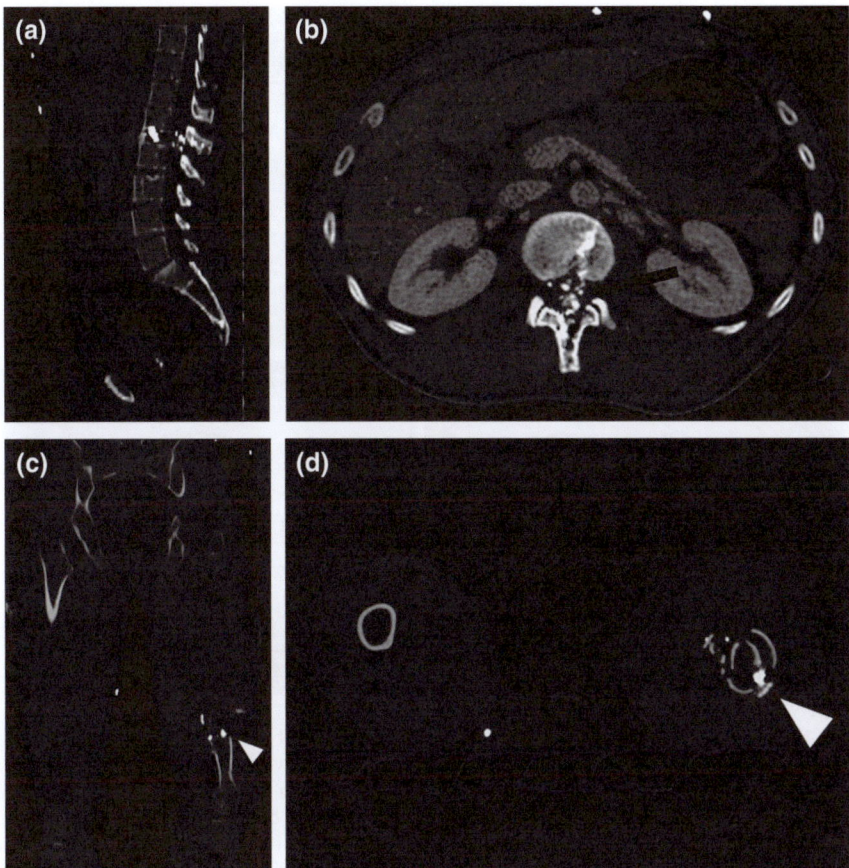

Fig. 12.2 A 28-year-old male victim of shooting with gunshot bullets locked in a lumbar vertebra and in left femur. **a** Sagittal MPR image shows a bullet locked at the L1–L2 intervertebral disk. **b** By impacting with the vertebral arch, the bullet has generated small metal and osseous fragments within the spinal canal causing an irreversible medulla damage (b, *arrow*). **c** Coronal MPR image and **d** axial scan show fracture of the femoral diaphysis caused by a further bullet that appears locked in the context of bone fragments (*arrowheads*)

Parietal hematomas, intra or extraluminal active bleeding (Fig. 12.3), and/or a focal wall thickening of a hollow viscus are also considered highly sensitive signs. The association with a mesenteric injury is not rare, manifesting as fat stranding or thickening, with or without active bleeding. Depending on the clinical context, nonoperative versus surgical or interventional approach with selective embolization should be selectively considered [27, 28].

Abdominal solid organs are often involved in penetrating traumas. Splenic injuries are more frequently associated to stab wounds, since majority of people is right-handed. Gunshot wounds in parenchymas are recognizable by the presence of

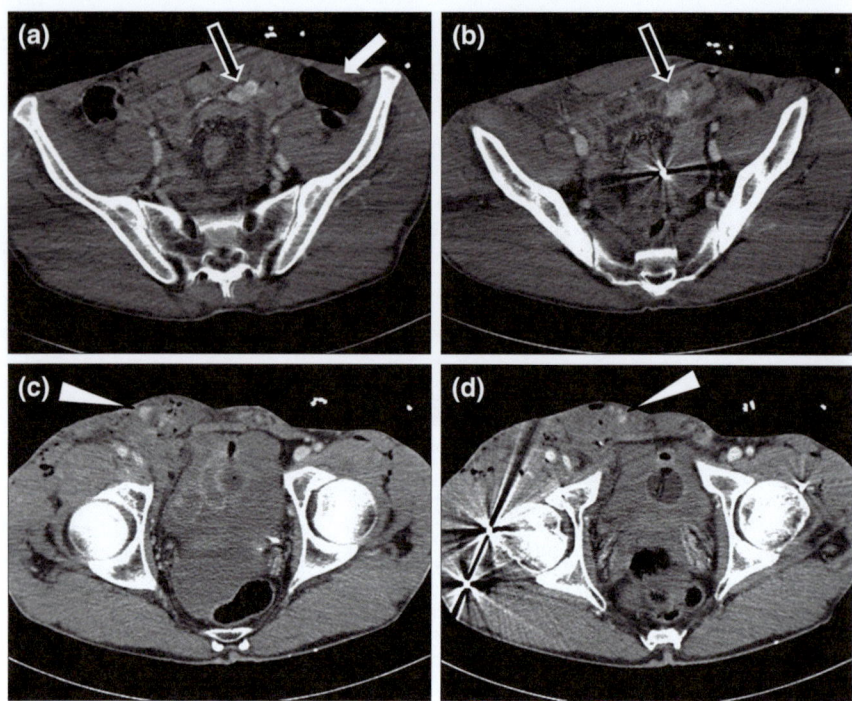

Fig. 12.3 A 42-year-old man with GI and groin injuries and active bleeding after birdshot wounds. **a, b** Two noncontiguous axial scans show foci of active bleeding in the pelvic cavity (*black arrows*) associated with an adjacent collection of free air in the left iliac fossa (a, *white arrow*) due to transmural injury on an ileal loop containing a birdshot bullet (**b**). **c, d** At the pelvis, two noncontiguous axial scans demonstrate hematoma of the right inguinal region, with mild subcutaneous emphysema and multiple foci of active bleeding (*arrowheads*). Furthermore, two birdshot bullets are visible in the contest on the right pelvic muscles (**d**)

a hypodense band of devascularization due to the transit of the projectile or a "cavity" due to tissue necrosis for the high temperature of the projectile. Sometimes a hollow space in the parenchyma persists over a time. Frequently in the context of parenchyma, vascular lesions such as foci of active bleeding, pseudoaneurysms, and/or arteriovenous fistulas are detectable [20].

In cases of renal injury after penetrating trauma, it is mandatory excluding foci of active bleeding and/or injuries at the excretory system, although very rarely the latter represent a priority in terms of immediate treatment (Fig. 12.4) [29].

In addition, MPR reformations are useful for evaluating the extent of tears, providing an additional viewpoint of any parenchymal injuries (Fig. 12.5).

Vascular injuries are diagnosed in the presence of active bleeding, pseudoaneurysms, arteriovenous fistulas or vascular occlusions. In these cases, selective embolization is the gold standard in terms of management approach [27].

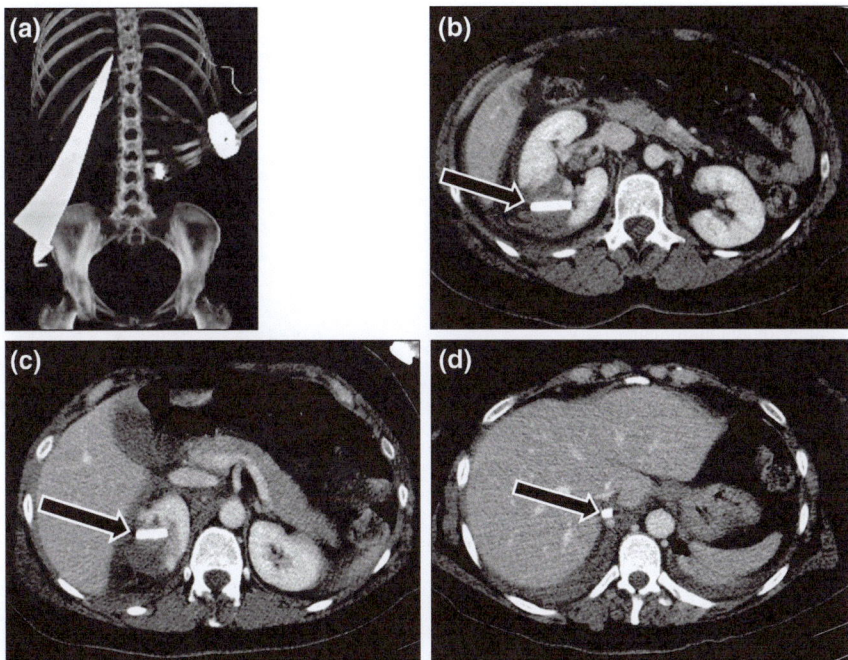

Fig. 12.4 A 35-year-old woman with deep retroperitoneal injury due to a blade of glass after a disastrous accidental fall into a window. **a** VR reconstruction image shows the presence of a huge glass splinter in the right flank. **b, c, d** Three noncontiguous axial scans show a deep laceration of the renal parenchyma with perirenal hematoma, due to the presence of a foreign body passing through the body in a caudal-cranial direction (*arrows*). **d** Note that the blade glass apex comes in close proximity with the retrohepatic inferior vena cava (*arrow*). No signs of retroperitoneal vessel laceration are visible. (*By courtesy of Dr. G. Casaburo, Department of Radiology, S. Paolo Hospital, Naples, Italy*)

A penetrating torso trauma should raise the suspicion of a diaphragmatic injury. Differently from blunt trauma, diaphragmatic tears due to stab wounds are smaller and not always clearly visible. The most specific radiological sign is represented by intrathoracic herniation of small amounts of abdominal fat or sub-diaphragmatic organs, with or without the presence of pathognomonic 'collar sign'. Other frequent CT findings of diaphragmatic injuries are the discontinuity of the diaphragm profile and the 'dependent viscera sign' [30]. In cases of impalement, it is easy to identify large diaphragmatic lacerations associated with evisceration of fat and abdominal organs below (Fig. 12.6).

Fig. 12.5 A 56-year-old man with stab wound in the lower thorax. **a** Patient's photograph at the admission. **b** CT scout view shows stab apex projecting at the level of a group of intestinal loops consistent with suspected intestinal perforation. **c** Sagittal MPR reformation image demonstrates the passage of the stab through the anterior diaphragmatic insertion, without colonic injury and/or free intraperitoneal air. After CT, the stab was removed and the patient was safely treated nonoperatively

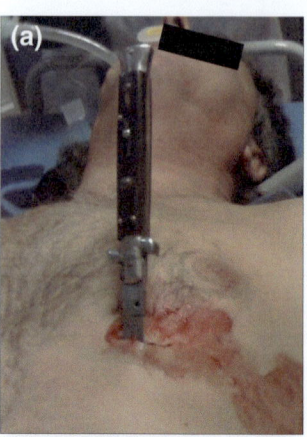
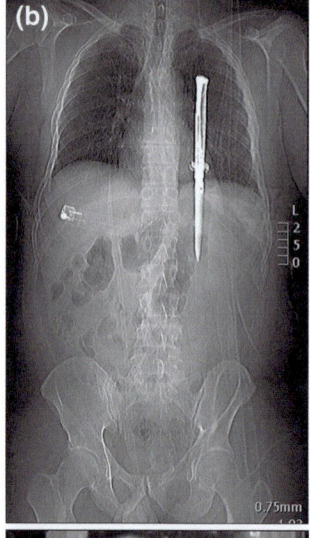
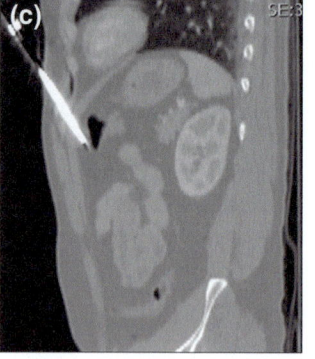

Fig. 12.6 A 68-year-old farmer victim of impalation, with left thoracoabdominal wall injury. **a** Patient's photograph at the admission showing evisceration of fat tissue after the penetrating injury. **b** Axial scan shows a huge laceration of left thoracoabdominal wall with evisceration of intra-abdominal fat. Note the large left emi-diaphragmatic tear with retraction and thickening of the diaphragmatic edges (*arrows*). **c** Coronal MPR clearly demonstrates the interruption of diaphragmatic profile (*arrow*) with intrathoracic herniation of abdominal content

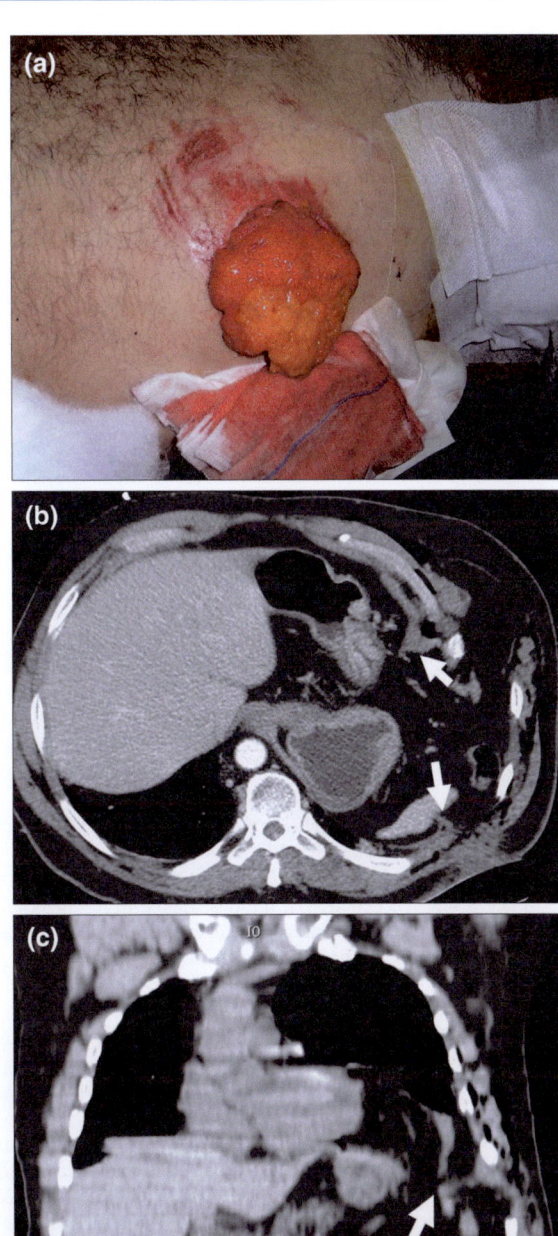

12.4 Conclusions

In case of penetrating wounds, the role of the radiologist relies on the early and definite characterization of injuries, thus directing the patient toward the most appropriate and timely management. In particular, CT examination allows early recognition of vascular, parenchymal and hollow viscera injuries, and detection of foreign bodies and its trajectory. At the same time, due to its high negative predictive value, CT can help select the patient that can be safely treated nonoperatively, reduce the number of unnecessary/nontherapeutic laparotomies, or guide toward a selective interventional approach.

References

1. Shaftan GW (1960) Indication for operation in abdominal trauma. Am J Surg 99:657–664
2. Feliciano DV, Burch JM, Spjut-Patrinely Y, Mattox KL, Jordan GL Jr, (1988) Abdominal gunshot wounds: an urban trauma center's experience with 300 consecutive patients. Ann Surg 208:362–370
3. Moore EE, Moore JB, Van Duzer-Moore S, Thompson JS. (1980) Mandatory laparotomy for gunshot wounds penetrating the abdomen. Am J Surg 140:847–851
4. Ivatury RR, Simon R, Stahl WM (1993) A critical evaluation of laparoscopy in penetrating abdominal trauma. J Trauma 34:822–828
5. Friedmann P (1968) Selective management of stab wounds of the abdomen. Arch Surg 96:292–295
6. Renz BM, Feliciano DV, (1995) Unnecessary laparotomies for trauma: a prospective study of morbidity. J Trauma 38:350–356
7. Fletcher TB, Setiawan H, Harrell RS et al (1989) Posterior abdominal stab wounds: role of CT evaluation. Radiology 173:621–625
8. Phillips T, Sclafani SA, Goldstein, et al (1986) Use of contrast-enhanced CT enema in the management of penetrating injuries trauma to the flank and back. J Trauma 26:593–600
9. Meyer DM, Thal ER, Weigelt JA et al (1989) The role of abdominal CT in the evaluation of stab wounds to the back. J trauma 29:1226–1230
10. Killeen KL, Shanmuganathan K, Poletti PA, Cooper C, Mirvis SE (2001) Helical computed tomography of bowel and mesenteric injuries. J Trauma 51:26–36
11. Butela ST, Federle MP, Chang PJ et al (2001) Performance of CT in detection of bowel injury. AJR 176:129–135
12. Himmelman RG, Martin M, Gilkey S et al (1991) Triple contrast CT scans in penetrating back and flank trauma. J Trauma 31:852–855
13. Kirton OC, Wint D, Thrasher B et al (1997) Stab wounds to the back and flank in the emodinamically stable patient: a decision algorithm based on contrast-enhanced computed tomography with colonic opacification. Am J Surg 173:189–193
14. Soto JA, Morales C, Munera F et al (2001) Penetrating stab wounds to the abdomen: use of serial US and contrast enhanced CT in stable patients. Radiology 220:365–371
15. Shanmuganathan K, Mirvis SE, Chiu WC et al (2004) Penetrating torso trauma: triple contrast helical CT in peritoneal violation and organ injury: a prospective study in 200 patients. Radiology 231:775–784
16. Ginzburg E, Carrillo EH, Kopelman T et al (1998) The role of computed tomography in selective management of gunshot wounds to the abdomen and flank. J Trauma 45:1005–1009
17. Feliciano DV, Burch JM, Spjut-Patrinely V et al (1988) Abdominal gunshot wounds. An urban trauma center's experience with 300 consecutive patients. Ann Surg 208:362–370

18. Munera F, Morales C, Soto JA et al (2004) Gunshot wounds of abdomen: evaluation of stable patients with triple contrast helical CT. Radiology 231:399–405
19. Velmahos GC, Constantinou C, Tillou A et al (2005) Abdominal computed tomographic scan for patients with gunshot wounds to the abdomen selected for nonoperative management. J Trauma 59:1155–1161
20. Castrillon GA, Soto JA (2012) Multidetector computed tomography of penetrating abdominal trauma. Semin Roentgenol 47:371–376
21. Woodruff JH Jr, Simonton JH (1959) Radiologic diagnosis in abdominal trauma. Calif Med 91:197–200
22. Mollberg NM, Wise SR, De Hoyos AL et al (2012) Chest computed tomography for penetrating thoracic trauma after normal screening chest roentgenogram. Ann Thorac Surg 93:1830–1835
23. Fry WR, Smith RS, Schnider JJ et al (1995) Ultrasonographic examination of the wound tract. Arch Surg 130:605–608
24. Ptak T, Rhea JT (2001) Novelline RA Experience with a continuous, single-pass whole body multi detector CT protocol for trauma: the three-minute multiple trauma CT scan. Emerg Radiol 8:250–56
25. Shanmuganathan K, Mirvis SE, Reaney SM (1995) Pictorial review: CT appearances of contrast medium extravasations associated with injury sustained from blunt abdominal trauma. Clin Radiol 50(3):182–187
26. Ramchandani P (2009) Buckler PM Imaging of genitourinary trauma. AJR Am J Roentgenol 192(6):1514–1523
27. Velmahos GC, Demetriades D, Chahwan S (1999) Angiographic embolization for arrest of bleeding after penetrating trauma to the abdomen. Am J Surg 178(5):367–373
28. Scaglione M, Romano L, Bocchini G et al (2012) Multidetector computed tomography of pancreatic, small bowel, and mesenteric traumas. Semin Roentgenol 47(4):362–370
29. Sica G, Bocchini G, Guida F et al (2010) Multidetector computed tomography in the diagnosis and management of renal trauma. Radiol Med 115(6):936–949
30. Bocchini G, Guida F, Sica G et al (2012) Diaphragmatic injuries after blunt trauma: are they still a challenge? reviewing CT findings and integrated imaging. Emerg Radiol 19(3):225–235

Index

A
Abdominal compartment syndrome, 47, 48
Abdominal ultrasound, 32
Abdominal wall meshes, 38, 39, 41, 44
Accidental ingestion, 25
Acute complications, 17
Adults, 1
Aluminum, 108
Arterial puncture, 83

B
Barium studies, 28
Battery ingestions, 29
Body packing, 31
Body stuffing, 31
Bowel obstruction, 34
Biliary obstruction, 63
Biliary tract, 55
Bullet wounds, 107

C
Catheter insertion, 82
Catheter perforation, 82
Central venous catheters, 81
Central venous thrombosis, 83
Cervical esophagus, 2
Checklist, 65
Children, 1, 27
Clinical history, 101
Complications, 56
Computed tomography (CT), 48, 111
Conventional radiography, 108

D
Damage control, 48
Devices, 62

Diagnostic problems, 31
Dislodged tubes, 55, 61

E
Elderly population, 61
Endoprostheses, 34, 56
Endoprosthetic stents, 84
Endovascular abdominal aortic aneurysm repair (EVAR), 84
Errors, 65
Esophagus, 27
Exogenous lipoid pneumonia, 16, 21

F
Fire-eater pneumonia, 16
Fish bones, 2
Food bolus impactions, 27
Foreign body, 1, 25, 105

G
Gastrografin, 28
Gastrointestinal, 25
Gastrointestinal stents, 61
Glass, 107
Gossypibomas, 38, 45

H
Hypopharyngeal foreign bodies, 27

I
Imaging techniques, 6
Ingestion, 1
Intravascular devices, 81
Intravascular foreign body, 81

L
Late complications, 17
Lentil aspiration pneumonia, 15, 20
Low-signal intensity, 102

M
Magnetic resonance (MR), 111
Magnetic resonance imaging (MRI), 32, 102
Mendelson's syndrome, 15, 20
Migration, 62
Multidetector row computed tomography (MDCT), 3, 25, 65
Multidetector row computed tomography angiography (MDCTA), 85
Multiorgan failure, 47

N
Near-drowning, 16
Near-drowning syndrome, 20
Neck, 7

O
Oropharynx, 2

P
Packing, 47–49, 51, 52
Patient management, 111
Perforation, 27, 29
Pharyngoesophageal FBs, 7
Plain abdominal X-ray, 32
Plain radiographic films, 85

R
Radiation hazard, 30
Radiography, 3, 25
Radiolucent foreign bodies, 111
Radio-opaque foreign bodies, 105
Radiopacity, 27
Radiopaque, 3
Radioscopy, 108
Rectal foreign bodies, 30
Retained, 105
Retained surgical foreign bodies, 37
Risk, 82
Rupture, 84

S
Scout MDCT, 30
Self-inserted soft-tissue foreign bodies, 106
Soft tissue, 105
Stent migration, 56
Stent obstruction, 56
Stents, 34, 55
Stomach, 28
Surrounding reactive lesion, 103
Surveillance post-EVAR, 85

T
Tract, 25

U
Ultrasonography, 108
Ultrasound-guided percutaneous removal, 111

MIX
Papier aus verantwortungsvollen Quellen
Paper from responsible sources
FSC® C105338

If you have any concerns about our products,
you can contact us on
ProductSafety@springernature.com

In case Publisher is established outside the EU,
the EU authorized representative is:
**Springer Nature Customer Service Center GmbH
Europaplatz 3, 69115 Heidelberg, Germany**

Printed by Libri Plureos GmbH
in Hamburg, Germany